# Introduction

Welcome to **"100+ Vegan Recipes for Managing Diverticulitis Flare-Up** comprehensive guide designed to support individuals navigating the challenges of diverticulitis while following a vegan lifestyle.

Diverticulitis, a condition characterized by inflamed pouches in the colon, can be uncomfortable and disruptive to daily life. Managing this condition often involves dietary adjustments to alleviate symptoms and promote digestive health. While traditional approaches may emphasize bland, low-fiber diets, this cookbook offers a fresh perspective by showcasing the diverse and flavorful world of vegan cuisine.

Our goal is to empower you to take control of your health and well-being through delicious, plant-based meals. Whether you're newly diagnosed or seeking new culinary inspiration on your journey with diverticulitis, this book is here to guide you. Each recipe has been carefully crafted with your needs in mind, focusing on ingredients that are gentle on the digestive system while providing essential nutrients and satisfying flavors.

In addition to the recipes, you'll find practical tips and guidance for managing diverticulitis through diet. We'll explore the importance of fiber, hydration, and gut-friendly ingredients, helping you make informed choices that support your digestive health.

With over 100 vegan recipes ranging from comforting soups and stews to vibrant salads and nourishing grain bowls, there's something for every palate and occasion. Whether you're craving a hearty meal to soothe symptoms during a flare-up or seeking light and refreshing options for everyday wellness, you'll find inspiration within these pages.

We believe that food should not only nourish the body but also delight the senses and bring joy to the table. By embracing the abundance of plant-based ingredients available to us, we can create meals that promote healing, vitality, and overall well-being.

Thank you for embarking on this culinary journey with us. Here's to delicious food, vibrant health, and thriving with diverticulitis.

# 1. Lentil soup

**Ingredients:**
- 1 cup dried brown or green lentils, rinsed
- 4 cups vegetable or chicken broth
- 1 onion, diced
- 2 carrots, peeled and diced
- 2 celery stalks, diced
- 3 garlic cloves, minced
- 1 tsp ground cumin
- 1 tsp dried thyme
- Salt and pepper to taste
- Chopped parsley for garnish (optional)

**Instructions:**

1. In a large pot, combine the lentils and broth. Bring to a boil over high heat.

2. Reduce heat to medium-low, cover and simmer for 15-20 minutes, until lentils are tender.

3. Add the onion, carrots, celery and garlic. Simmer for 10-15 minutes more, until vegetables are soft.

4. Stir in the cumin, thyme, salt and pepper.

5. Taste and adjust seasonings as needed.

6. Serve hot, garnished with chopped parsley if desired.

This makes a hearty, comforting lentil soup that's packed with fiber, protein and veggies. Enjoy!

# 2. Vegetable stir-fry with tofu

**Ingredients**:
- 1 block (14 oz) extra-firm tofu, pressed and cubed
- 2 tbsp vegetable or peanut oil
- 2 cups mixed vegetables (such as broccoli, bell peppers, snap peas, carrots, mushrooms)
- 3 cloves garlic, minced
- 1 tbsp grated fresh ginger
- 2 tbsp low-sodium soy sauce
- 1 tbsp rice vinegar or lime juice
- 1 tsp sesame oil
- Salt and pepper to taste
- Cooked rice or noodles, for serving

**Instructions**:

1. In a large skillet or wok, heat the 2 tbsp of oil over medium-high heat. Add the cubed tofu and cook for 5-7 minutes, turning occasionally, until lightly browned on all sides. Transfer tofu to a plate.

2. In the same pan, add the mixed vegetables and stir-fry for 3-5 minutes until starting to soften.

3. Add the garlic and ginger and cook for 1 minute more, until fragrant.

4. Return the tofu to the pan. Pour in the soy sauce, rice vinegar/lime juice, and sesame oil. Toss everything together and cook for 2-3 minutes more.

5. Season with salt and pepper to taste.

6. Serve the stir-fry immediately over steamed rice or noodles. Enjoy!

***You can customize the vegetables based on what's in season or your preferences. This makes a quick, healthy and flavorful vegetarian meal.***

# 3. Quinoa salad with roasted vegetables

**Ingredients**:
- 1 cup uncooked quinoa, rinsed
- 2 cups vegetable or chicken broth
- 1 medium zucchini, diced
- 1 red bell pepper, diced
- 1 cup cherry tomatoes, halved
- 1 red onion, diced
- 2 tbsp olive oil
- Salt and pepper to taste
- 2 tbsp chopped fresh parsley
- 2 tbsp crumbled feta cheese (optional)

*For the Dressing:*
- 2 tbsp olive oil
- 2 tbsp lemon juice
- 1 tsp Dijon mustard
- 1 tsp honey
- Salt and pepper to taste

**Instructions:**

1. Preheat oven to 400°F. Toss the diced zucchini, bell pepper, and onion with 2 tbsp olive oil on a baking sheet. Season with salt and pepper. Roast for 20-25 minutes, until vegetables are tender and lightly browned.

2. Meanwhile, in a medium saucepan, combine the quinoa and broth. Bring to a boil, then reduce heat to low, cover and simmer for 15-20 minutes, until quinoa is cooked through. Fluff with a fork and let cool slightly.

3. In a large bowl, combine the cooked quinoa, roasted vegetables, and cherry tomatoes.

4. In a small bowl, whisk together the dressing ingredients - olive oil, lemon juice, mustard, honey, salt and pepper.

5. Pour the dressing over the quinoa salad and toss to coat. Sprinkle with chopped parsley and crumbled feta (if using). Serve chilled or at room temperature. Enjoy!

**This quinoa salad is packed with nutritious veggies and makes a great side dish or light main course.**

# 4. Chickpea curry

**Ingredients:**
- 2 tbsp olive oil
- 1 onion, diced
- 3 cloves garlic, minced
- 1 tbsp grated fresh ginger
- 2 tsp garam masala
- 1 tsp ground cumin
- 1 tsp ground coriander
- 1 tsp turmeric
- 1/4 tsp cayenne pepper (or to taste)
- 1 (15oz) can diced tomatoes
- 1 (15oz) can chickpeas, drained and rinsed
- 1 cup vegetable or chicken broth
- 1 cup coconut milk
- Salt and pepper to taste
- Chopped cilantro for garnish

**Instructions:**
1. In a large skillet or pot, heat the olive oil over medium heat. Add the diced onion and sauté for 5-7 minutes until translucent.

2. Add the garlic and ginger and cook for 1 minute, until fragrant.

3. Stir in the garam masala, cumin, coriander, turmeric and cayenne. Cook for 2 minutes to toast the spices.

4. Pour in the diced tomatoes, chickpeas, broth and coconut milk. Bring to a simmer.

5. Reduce heat to medium-low and let the curry simmer for 15-20 minutes, until thickened slightly.

6. Season with salt and pepper to taste.

7. Serve the chickpea curry over basmati rice or with naan bread. Garnish with chopped cilantro.

*This curry is packed with protein from the chickpeas and has a rich, creamy coconut milk base. It's a delicious vegetarian main dish.*

# 5. Black bean soup

**Ingredients:**
- 2 tbsp olive oil
- 1 onion, diced
- 3 cloves garlic, minced
- 2 carrots, peeled and diced
- 2 celery stalks, diced
- 2 tsp ground cumin
- 1 tsp dried oregano
- 1/4 tsp cayenne pepper (or to taste)
- 2 (15oz) cans black beans, drained and rinsed
- 4 cups vegetable or chicken broth
- 1 (15oz) can diced tomatoes
- Salt and pepper to taste
- Chopped cilantro, sour cream, and lime wedges for serving

**Instructions:**

1. In a large pot or Dutch oven, heat the olive oil over medium heat. Add the onion and sauté for 5 minutes until translucent.

2. Add the garlic, carrots, and celery. Cook for 3-4 minutes, stirring frequently, until vegetables start to soften.

3. Stir in the cumin, oregano, and cayenne. Cook for 1 minute to toast the spices.

4. Add the black beans, broth, and diced tomatoes. Bring to a simmer.

5. Reduce heat to medium-low and let the soup simmer for 20-25 minutes, until the vegetables are very tender.

6. Use an immersion blender or regular blender to puree about half of the soup, leaving some beans and vegetables intact.

7. Season with salt and pepper to taste.

8. Serve the black bean soup hot, garnished with chopped cilantro, a dollop of sour cream, and a squeeze of fresh lime juice.

**This hearty, flavorful black bean soup is delicious on its own or with cornbread or tortilla chips on the side.**

# 6. Ratatouille

**Ingredients:**
- 2 tbsp olive oil
- 1 medium eggplant, diced
- 1 zucchini, diced
- 1 yellow squash, diced
- 1 red bell pepper, diced
- 1 onion, diced
- 3 cloves garlic, minced
- 1 (14oz) can diced tomatoes
- 2 tbsp tomato paste
- 1 tsp dried thyme
- 1 tsp dried oregano
- Salt and pepper to taste
- Chopped fresh basil for garnish

**Instructions:**

1. In a large skillet or Dutch oven, heat the olive oil over medium heat. Add the diced eggplant, zucchini, squash, bell pepper, and onion. Sauté for 8-10 minutes, stirring occasionally, until vegetables are starting to soften.

2. Add the minced garlic and cook for 1 minute more, until fragrant.

3. Stir in the diced tomatoes, tomato paste, thyme, oregano, and a pinch each of salt and pepper.

4. Bring the mixture to a simmer, then reduce heat to medium-low. Let the ratatouille simmer for 20-25 minutes, stirring occasionally, until the vegetables are very tender.

5. Taste and adjust seasoning as needed, adding more salt, pepper, or herbs to your preference.

6. Serve the ratatouille warm, garnished with chopped fresh basil. It can be enjoyed on its own or served over pasta, rice, or crusty bread.

*This classic French vegetable stew is full of fresh, summery flavors. The long simmer allows the flavors to meld together beautifully.*

# 7. Lentil stew

**Ingredients:**
- 2 tbsp olive oil
- 1 onion, diced
- 3 carrots, peeled and diced
- 3 celery stalks, diced
- 4 cloves garlic, minced
- 1 lb brown or green lentils, rinsed
- 6 cups vegetable or chicken broth
- 1 (14oz) can diced tomatoes
- 2 tsp dried thyme
- 1 tsp smoked paprika
- Salt and pepper to taste
- Chopped parsley for garnish

**Instructions:**

1. In a large pot or Dutch oven, heat the olive oil over medium heat. Add the diced onion, carrots, and celery. Sauté for 5-7 minutes until the vegetables start to soften.

2. Add the minced garlic and cook for 1 minute more, until fragrant.

3. Stir in the rinsed lentils, broth, diced tomatoes, thyme, and smoked paprika. Season with salt and pepper.

4. Bring the stew to a boil, then reduce heat to medium-low. Simmer for 25-30 minutes, stirring occasionally, until the lentils are very tender.

5. Taste and adjust seasoning as needed, adding more salt, pepper, or herbs to your preference.

6. Serve the lentil stew hot, garnished with chopped fresh parsley. It's delicious on its own or with crusty bread.

***This hearty, protein-packed lentil stew is perfect for a cozy meal. The smoked paprika adds a nice depth of flavor.***

# 8. Vegetable fajitas with guacamole

*For the Fajitas:*
- 2 tbsp olive oil
- 1 red bell pepper, sliced
- 1 yellow bell pepper, sliced
- 1 red onion, sliced
- 8 oz mushrooms, sliced
- 2 tsp chili powder
- 1 tsp ground cumin
- 1 tsp garlic powder
- Salt and pepper to taste
- 8-10 small flour or corn tortillas, warmed

*For the Guacamole:*
- 2 ripe avocados, pitted and diced
- 1 Roma tomato, diced
- 1/4 cup diced red onion
- 1 jalapeño, seeded and minced (optional)
- 2 tbsp chopped cilantro
- 1 tbsp lime juice
- 1/4 tsp salt

## Instructions:

1. Make the guacamole: In a medium bowl, gently mix together the diced avocado, tomato, onion, jalapeño (if using), cilantro, lime juice and salt. Set aside.

2. In a large skillet or wok, heat the olive oil over medium-high heat. Add the sliced bell peppers, onion and mushrooms. Sauté for 5-7 minutes until vegetables are tender-crisp.

3. Sprinkle the vegetables with the chili powder, cumin, garlic powder, salt and pepper. Toss to coat evenly.

4. Serve the sautéed vegetables in the warmed tortillas, topped with a generous spoonful of the fresh guacamole.

5. Provide any additional desired toppings like shredded cheese, sour cream, salsa, etc.

*These veggie fajitas make a delicious, healthy meatless meal. The homemade guacamole adds a creamy, flavorful topping.*

# 9. Lentil salad with lemon vinaigrette

***For the Salad:***
- 1 cup uncooked brown or green lentils, rinsed
- 3 cups vegetable or chicken broth
- 1 cucumber, diced
- 1 cup cherry tomatoes, halved
- 1/2 red onion, thinly sliced
- 1/4 cup crumbled feta cheese
- 2 tbsp chopped fresh parsley

***For the Lemon Vinaigrette:***
- 3 tbsp olive oil
- 2 tbsp lemon juice
- 1 tsp Dijon mustard
- 1 tsp honey
- 1 garlic clove, minced
- Salt and pepper to taste

**Instructions:**

1. In a medium saucepan, combine the lentils and broth. Bring to a boil, then reduce heat to medium-low, cover and simmer for 15-20 minutes, until lentils are tender. Drain and let cool.

2. In a large bowl, combine the cooked lentils, diced cucumber, halved tomatoes, sliced red onion, crumbled feta, and chopped parsley.

3. In a small bowl, whisk together the olive oil, lemon juice, Dijon mustard, honey, and minced garlic. Season with salt and pepper.

4. Pour the lemon vinaigrette over the lentil salad and toss gently to coat.

5. Refrigerate the salad for at least 30 minutes to allow the flavors to meld.

6. Serve chilled or at room temperature. Enjoy!

**This bright, refreshing lentil salad makes a great side dish or light main course. The lemon vinaigrette adds a nice tangy flavor.**

# 10. Roasted vegetable medley

**Ingredients:**
- 1 lb Brussels sprouts, trimmed and halved
- 2 carrots, peeled and cut into 1-inch pieces
- 1 red bell pepper, cut into 1-inch pieces
- 1 zucchini, cut into 1-inch pieces
- 1 red onion, cut into 1-inch wedges
- 3 tbsp olive oil
- 2 tsp dried thyme
- 1 tsp garlic powder
- Salt and pepper to taste
- Chopped parsley for garnish (optional)

**Instructions:**

1. Preheat oven to 400°F. Line a large baking sheet with parchment paper.

2. In a large bowl, toss the Brussels sprouts, carrots, bell pepper, zucchini, and onion with the olive oil, thyme, garlic powder, salt and pepper until evenly coated.

3. Spread the vegetables out in a single layer on the prepared baking sheet.

4. Roast for 25-30 minutes, flipping the vegetables halfway, until they are tender and starting to caramelize.

5. Remove the roasted vegetables from the oven and transfer to a serving bowl.

6. Garnish with chopped fresh parsley if desired.

7. Serve the roasted vegetable medley warm or at room temperature. It makes a great side dish or can be enjoyed on its own.

**You can easily customize this recipe by using different seasonal vegetables. The key is to cut them into similar-sized pieces so they cook evenly. Enjoy this flavorful, healthy roasted veggie dish!**

# 11. Vegetarian chili

**Ingredients**:
- 2 tbsp olive oil
- 1 onion, diced
- 3 cloves garlic, minced
- 2 bell peppers (any color), diced
- 2 carrots, peeled and diced
- 2 celery stalks, diced
- 2 (15oz) cans black beans, drained and rinsed
- 2 (15oz) cans kidney beans, drained and rinsed
- 1 (15oz) can diced tomatoes
- 1 (6oz) can tomato paste
- 2 tbsp chili powder
- 2 tsp ground cumin
- 1 tsp dried oregano
- 1 tsp smoked paprika
- 1/4 tsp cayenne pepper (or to taste)
- Salt and pepper to taste
- Chopped cilantro, shredded cheese, sour cream for serving

**Instructions**:
1. In a large pot or Dutch oven, heat the olive oil over medium heat. Add the diced onion and sauté for 5-7 minutes until translucent.

2. Add the minced garlic, bell peppers, carrots, and celery. Cook for 3-4 minutes, stirring frequently, until vegetables start to soften.

3. Stir in the black beans, kidney beans, diced tomatoes, tomato paste, chili powder, cumin, oregano, smoked paprika, and cayenne. Season with salt and pepper.

4. Bring the chili to a simmer, then reduce heat to medium-low. Let it simmer for 20-25 minutes, stirring occasionally, until thickened.

5. Taste and adjust seasonings as needed, adding more spices, salt or pepper to your taste.

6. Serve the vegetarian chili hot, garnished with chopped cilantro, shredded cheese, and a dollop of sour cream.

**This hearty, protein-packed chili is delicious on its own or served with cornbread, tortilla chips or crusty bread. It's a satisfying meatless meal.**

# 12. Cauliflower fried rice

**Ingredients**:
- 1 head of cauliflower, cut into florets
- 2 tbsp sesame oil
- 1 onion, diced
- 2 carrots, peeled and diced
- 1 cup frozen peas
- 3 cloves garlic, minced
- 1 tbsp grated fresh ginger
- 2 eggs, lightly beaten
- 3 tbsp low-sodium soy sauce
- 1 tsp sesame oil
- Salt and pepper to taste
- Chopped green onions for garnish

**Instructions**:

1. In a food processor, pulse the cauliflower florets until they are broken down into small, rice-like pieces. Set aside.

2. In a large skillet or wok, heat 2 tbsp sesame oil over medium-high heat. Add the diced onion and carrots. Sauté for 3-4 minutes until starting to soften.

3. Add the frozen peas, minced garlic, and grated ginger. Cook for 1 minute more, until fragrant.

4. Push the vegetables to the side of the pan. Pour the beaten eggs into the empty space and let them cook for 30 seconds to 1 minute, then scramble them.

5. Add the riced cauliflower to the pan and stir everything together. Cook for 5-7 minutes, stirring frequently, until the cauliflower is tender.

6. Drizzle the soy sauce and 1 tsp sesame oil over the cauliflower fried rice. Toss to coat evenly.

7. Season with salt and pepper to taste.

8. Serve the cauliflower fried rice hot, garnished with chopped green onions.

**This healthy, veggie-packed fried rice makes a great meatless main dish or side. The cauliflower provides a low-carb alternative to traditional rice.**

# 13. Tofu stir-fry with broccoli and carrots

**Ingredients:**
- 1 block (14 oz) extra-firm tofu, pressed and cubed
- 2 tbsp vegetable or peanut oil
- 3 cups broccoli florets
- 2 carrots, peeled and sliced
- 3 cloves garlic, minced
- 1 tbsp grated fresh ginger
- 2 tbsp low-sodium soy sauce
- 1 tbsp rice vinegar
- 1 tsp sesame oil
- Salt and pepper to taste
- Cooked rice, for serving

**Instructions:**

1. In a large skillet or wok, heat the 2 tbsp of oil over medium-high heat. Add the cubed tofu and cook for 5-7 minutes, turning occasionally, until lightly browned on all sides. Transfer tofu to a plate.

2. In the same pan, add the broccoli florets and sliced carrots. Stir-fry for 4-5 minutes until starting to soften.

3. Add the minced garlic and grated ginger. Cook for 1 minute more, until fragrant.

4. Return the cooked tofu to the pan. Pour in the soy sauce, rice vinegar, and sesame oil. Toss everything together and cook for 2-3 minutes more.

5. Season with salt and pepper to taste.

6. Serve the tofu stir-fry immediately over steamed rice. Enjoy!

***You can customize the vegetables based on your preferences. This makes a quick, healthy and flavorful vegetarian meal.***

# 14. Lentil shepherd's pie

**For the Filling:**
- 1 cup dry brown or green lentils, rinsed
- 4 cups vegetable or chicken broth
- 1 tbsp olive oil
- 1 onion, diced
- 3 carrots, peeled and diced
- 3 celery stalks, diced
- 3 cloves garlic, minced
- 2 tsp dried thyme
- 1 tsp dried rosemary
- 1 (15oz) can diced tomatoes
- Salt and pepper to taste

**For the Topping:**
- 3 lbs russet or Yukon Gold potatoes, peeled and cut into 1-inch chunks
- 1/4 cup milk
- 2 tbsp butter
- 1/2 cup shredded cheddar cheese (optional)

**Instructions**:
1. Preheat oven to 375°F.

2. In a medium saucepan, combine the lentils and broth. Bring to a boil, then reduce heat and simmer for 20-25 minutes, until lentils are tender. Drain any excess liquid.

3. In a large skillet, heat the olive oil over medium heat. Add the onion, carrots, and celery. Sauté for 5-7 minutes until starting to soften.

4. Stir in the minced garlic, thyme, and rosemary. Cook for 1 minute more.

5. Add the cooked lentils and diced tomatoes. Season with salt and pepper. Simmer for 5 minutes.

6. Meanwhile, in a large pot, cover the potato chunks with water and bring to a boil. Cook for 15-20 minutes until very tender. Drain and mash with the milk and butter.

7. Spread the lentil filling into a 9x13 baking dish. Top with the mashed potatoes, smoothing them evenly over the top.

8. If using, sprinkle the shredded cheddar over the potatoes. Bake for 25-30 minutes, until the potatoes are lightly browned. Let stand for 5 minutes before serving.

*This hearty lentil shepherd's pie makes a delicious meatless main dish. The creamy mashed potato topping is the perfect complement to the savory lentil filling.*

# 15. Vegetable curry with coconut milk

**Ingredients:**
- 2 tbsp coconut oil or olive oil
- 1 onion, diced
- 3 cloves garlic, minced
- 1 tbsp grated fresh ginger
- 2 tsp garam masala
- 1 tsp ground cumin
- 1 tsp ground coriander
- 1/4 tsp cayenne pepper (or to taste)
- 1 medium sweet potato, peeled and cubed
- 1 cup cauliflower florets
- 1 cup green beans, trimmed and cut into 1-inch pieces
- 1 (13.5 oz) can full-fat coconut milk
- 1 cup vegetable or chicken broth
- 1 tsp salt
- Chopped cilantro for garnish
- Cooked basmati rice, for serving

**Instructions:**

1. In a large skillet or Dutch oven, heat the coconut oil over medium heat. Add the diced onion and sauté for 5-7 minutes until translucent.

2. Stir in the minced garlic and grated ginger. Cook for 1 minute until fragrant.

3. Add the garam masala, cumin, coriander, and cayenne. Cook for 2 minutes to toast the spices.

4. Add the cubed sweet potato, cauliflower florets, and green beans. Stir to coat the vegetables in the spices.

5. Pour in the coconut milk and vegetable broth. Season with 1 tsp salt.

6. Bring the curry to a simmer, then reduce heat to medium-low. Let it simmer for 20-25 minutes, until the vegetables are very tender.

7. Taste and adjust seasoning as needed, adding more salt, pepper, or spices to your preference.

8. Serve the vegetable curry over steamed basmati rice, garnished with chopped fresh cilantro.

# 16. Quinoa tabbouleh

**ngredients:**
- 1 cup uncooked quinoa, rinsed
- 2 cups vegetable or chicken broth
- 1 cup diced cucumber
- 1 cup halved cherry tomatoes
- 1/2 cup diced red onion
- 1/2 cup chopped fresh parsley
- 1/4 cup chopped fresh mint
- 2 tbsp olive oil
- 2 tbsp lemon juice
- 1 tsp Dijon mustard
- 1 garlic clove, minced
- Salt and pepper to taste

**Instructions:**

1. In a medium saucepan, combine the quinoa and broth. Bring to a boil, then reduce heat to low, cover and simmer for 15-20 minutes, until quinoa is cooked through. Fluff with a fork and let cool.

2. In a large bowl, combine the cooked quinoa, diced cucumber, halved cherry tomatoes, diced red onion, chopped parsley, and chopped mint.

3. In a small bowl, whisk together the olive oil, lemon juice, Dijon mustard, and minced garlic. Season with salt and pepper.

4. Pour the dressing over the quinoa salad and toss gently to coat.

5. Refrigerate the tabbouleh for at least 30 minutes to allow the flavors to meld.

6. Serve chilled or at room temperature. Enjoy!

*This fresh, herby quinoa tabbouleh makes a great side dish or light main course. The quinoa provides protein and fiber, while the vegetables and herbs give it a bright, refreshing flavor.*

# 17. Stuffed mushrooms with spinach and breadcrumbs

**Ingredients:**
- 16 oz cremini or button mushrooms, stems removed and finely chopped
- 2 tbsp olive oil
- 1/2 onion, finely diced
- 2 cloves garlic, minced
- 5 oz fresh spinach, chopped
- 1/4 cup panko breadcrumbs
- 1/4 cup grated Parmesan cheese
- 2 tbsp cream cheese, softened
- 1 tsp dried thyme
- Salt and pepper to taste

**Instructions:**

1. Preheat oven to 375°F. Clean the mushrooms and remove the stems, finely chopping the stems.

2. In a skillet, heat the olive oil over medium heat. Add the chopped mushroom stems, diced onion, and minced garlic. Sauté for 5-7 minutes until softened.

3. Add the chopped spinach and cook for 2-3 minutes more, until the spinach is wilted. Remove from heat and let cool slightly.

4. In a medium bowl, combine the sautéed mushroom mixture, panko breadcrumbs, Parmesan cheese, cream cheese, and dried thyme. Season with salt and pepper.

5. Stuff the mushroom caps evenly with the spinach-breadcrumb filling.

6. Arrange the stuffed mushrooms on a baking sheet. Bake for 15-18 minutes, until the mushrooms are tender and the filling is hot.

7. Serve the stuffed mushrooms warm. Enjoy!

***These cheesy, breadcrumb-topped stuffed mushrooms make a delicious appetizer or side dish. The spinach adds a nice fresh flavor.***

# 18. Veggie sushi rolls with avocado and cucumber

**Ingredients**:
- 1 cup uncooked short-grain sushi rice
- 2 tbsp rice vinegar
- 1 tsp sugar
- 1/2 tsp salt
- 1 avocado, sliced
- 1 cucumber, peeled and cut into thin strips
- 1 carrot, peeled and cut into thin strips
- 1 red bell pepper, cut into thin strips
- 4-6 sheets nori (seaweed sheets)
- Soy sauce, pickled ginger, and wasabi for serving

**Instructions:**

1. Cook the sushi rice according to package instructions. Transfer to a large bowl and stir in the rice vinegar, sugar, and salt. Let cool completely.

2. Lay a sheet of nori on a bamboo sushi mat or clean surface. Spread about 3/4 cup of the cooled sushi rice evenly over the nori, leaving a 1-inch border at the top.

3. Arrange a few slices of avocado, cucumber, carrot, and red pepper in a line across the center of the rice.

4. Carefully lift the bottom edge of the sushi mat and roll it tightly over the filling, using the mat to shape the roll. Moisten the top edge of the nori with water to seal the roll.

5. Repeat with the remaining nori sheets and fillings to make 4-6 rolls total.

6. Using a very sharp knife, slice each roll into 6-8 pieces.

7. Serve the veggie sushi rolls immediately with soy sauce, pickled ginger, and wasabi on the side for dipping.

***These fresh, colorful veggie sushi rolls make a delicious and healthy appetizer or light meal. The creamy avocado and crunchy vegetables are a tasty combination.***

# 19. Roasted Brussels sprouts with balsamic glaze

**Ingredients:**
- 1 lb Brussels sprouts, trimmed and halved
- 2 tbsp olive oil
- Salt and pepper to taste
- 2 tbsp balsamic vinegar
- 1 tbsp honey
- 1 tsp Dijon mustard
- 1 garlic clove, minced
- Chopped parsley for garnish (optional)

**Instructions:**

1. Preheat oven to 400°F. Line a baking sheet with parchment paper.

2. In a large bowl, toss the trimmed and halved Brussels sprouts with the olive oil. Season with salt and pepper.

3. Spread the Brussels sprouts in a single layer on the prepared baking sheet.

4. Roast for 20-25 minutes, flipping halfway, until the sprouts are tender and lightly browned.

5. In a small bowl, whisk together the balsamic vinegar, honey, Dijon mustard, and minced garlic.

6. Transfer the roasted Brussels sprouts to a serving bowl. Drizzle the balsamic glaze over the top and toss to coat evenly.

7. Garnish with chopped fresh parsley if desired.

8. Serve the roasted Brussels sprouts warm. Enjoy!

***The balsamic glaze adds a sweet and tangy flavor that complements the roasted Brussels sprouts perfectly. This makes a delicious side dish.***

# 20. Tofu lettuce wraps

**Ingredients**:
- 1 block (14 oz) extra-firm tofu, pressed and crumbled
- 2 tbsp soy sauce
- 1 tbsp rice vinegar
- 1 tsp sesame oil
- 1 tbsp vegetable oil
- 3 cloves garlic, minced
- 1 tbsp grated fresh ginger
- 1 cup shredded carrots
- 1 cup thinly sliced mushrooms
- 1/2 cup diced water chestnuts
- 2 tbsp chopped green onions
- 1 head butter or romaine lettuce, leaves separated

*For the Sauce:*
- 2 tbsp hoisin sauce
- 1 tbsp rice vinegar
- 1 tsp sesame oil
- 1 tsp Sriracha or other hot sauce (optional)

**Instructions:**

1. In a medium bowl, combine the crumbled tofu, soy sauce, rice vinegar, and 1 tsp sesame oil. Toss to coat the tofu.

2. In a large skillet or wok, heat the 1 tbsp vegetable oil over medium-high heat. Add the minced garlic and grated ginger. Cook for 1 minute until fragrant.

3. Add the seasoned tofu to the pan and cook for 5-7 minutes, stirring occasionally, until lightly browned.

4. Stir in the shredded carrots, sliced mushrooms, diced water chestnuts, and chopped green onions. Cook for 2-3 minutes more.

5. In a small bowl, whisk together the ingredients for the sauce - hoisin, rice vinegar, sesame oil, and Sriracha (if using).

6. To serve, place a spoonful of the tofu mixture into a lettuce leaf. Drizzle with the hoisin sauce. Enjoy the tofu lettuce wraps immediately.

*These fresh, flavorful tofu lettuce wraps make a delicious and healthy meatless meal or appetizer. The crunchy veggies and savory sauce are a winning combination.*

# 21. Chickpea salad with cucumber and tomatoes

**Ingredients:**
- 2 (15oz) cans chickpeas, drained and rinsed
- 1 cucumber, diced
- 1 pint cherry or grape tomatoes, halved
- 1/2 red onion, thinly sliced
- 1/4 cup chopped fresh parsley
- 2 tbsp olive oil
- 2 tbsp lemon juice
- 1 tsp Dijon mustard
- 1 garlic clove, minced
- Salt and pepper to taste

**Instructions:**

1. In a large bowl, combine the drained and rinsed chickpeas, diced cucumber, halved tomatoes, sliced red onion, and chopped parsley.

2. In a small bowl, whisk together the olive oil, lemon juice, Dijon mustard, and minced garlic. Season with salt and pepper.

3. Pour the dressing over the chickpea salad and toss gently to coat.

4. Cover and refrigerate the salad for at least 30 minutes to allow the flavors to meld.

5. Serve chilled or at room temperature. This chickpea salad makes a great side dish or light main course.

You can customize the vegetables based on what's fresh and in season. The lemon-Dijon dressing provides a bright, tangy flavor that complements the chickpeas and veggies.

***This protein-packed salad is perfect for a healthy lunch or dinner. Enjoy!***

# 22. Broccoli and cheddar quiche (using vegan cheese)

*Crust:*
- 1 1/4 cups all-purpose flour
- 1/2 tsp salt
- 1/3 cup cold vegan butter, cubed
- 3-4 tbsp ice water

*Filling*:
- 1 head broccoli, cut into small florets
- 1 tbsp olive oil
- 1 onion, diced
- 3 cloves garlic, minced
- 1 cup unsweetened almond milk
- 1/2 cup vegan cheddar cheese, shredded
- 1/4 cup nutritional yeast
- 1 tsp Dijon mustard
- 1/2 tsp dried thyme
- 1/4 tsp cayenne pepper
- Salt and pepper to taste
- 3 eggs or 3 tbsp aquafaba (chickpea liquid)

**Instructions**:
1. Make the crust: In a food processor, pulse the flour and salt. Add the cold vegan butter and pulse until mixture resembles coarse crumbs. Add ice water 1 tbsp at a time, pulsing until dough just begins to hold together. Form dough into a disc, wrap in plastic and refrigerate for 30 minutes.

2. Preheat oven to 375°F. Roll out the chilled dough and press into a 9-inch pie dish. Prick the bottom with a fork. Bake for 12-15 minutes until lightly golden.

3. For the filling, steam the broccoli florets until tender-crisp, about 5 minutes. Drain and set aside.

4. In a skillet, heat the olive oil over medium heat. Add the diced onion and sauté for 5 minutes until translucent. Add the minced garlic and cook for 1 minute more.

5. In a blender, combine the almond milk, vegan cheddar, nutritional yeast, Dijon, thyme, cayenne, salt and pepper. Blend until smooth.

6. In a large bowl, whisk the eggs (or aquafaba). Slowly whisk in the blended milk mixture.

7. Arrange the steamed broccoli in the pre-baked pie crust. Pour the egg mixture over top.

8. Bake for 35-40 minutes, until the center is set. Let cool for 10 minutes before slicing.

**This vegan broccoli cheddar quiche is a delicious meatless option. The creamy, cheesy filling pairs perfectly with the flaky crust.**

# 23. Tofu tikka masala

**Ingredients:**
- 1 block (14 oz) extra-firm tofu, pressed and cubed
- 2 tbsp olive oil
- 1 onion, diced
- 3 cloves garlic, minced
- 1 tbsp grated fresh ginger
- 2 tsp garam masala
- 1 tsp ground cumin
- 1 tsp paprika
- 1/4 tsp cayenne pepper (or to taste)
- 1 (15 oz) can diced tomatoes
- 1 cup coconut milk
- 1 tbsp tomato paste
- 1 tsp sugar
- Salt and pepper to taste
- Chopped cilantro for garnish
- Cooked basmati rice, for serving

**Instructions:**

1. In a large skillet or wok, heat the 2 tbsp of olive oil over medium-high heat. Add the cubed tofu and cook for 5-7 minutes, turning occasionally, until lightly browned on all sides. Transfer tofu to a plate.

2. In the same pan, add the diced onion and sauté for 5 minutes until translucent.

3. Stir in the minced garlic and grated ginger. Cook for 1 minute more, until fragrant.

4. Add the garam masala, cumin, paprika, and cayenne. Cook for 2 minutes to toast the spices.

5. Pour in the diced tomatoes, coconut milk, tomato paste, and sugar. Stir to combine.

6. Gently fold the cooked tofu back into the sauce. Simmer for 10-15 minutes, until the sauce has thickened.

7. Season with salt and pepper to taste.

8. Serve the tofu tikka masala immediately over steamed basmati rice, garnished with chopped fresh cilantro.

**This creamy, flavorful tofu tikka masala makes a delicious vegetarian main dish. The tofu soaks up all the aromatic spices.**

# 24. Spinach and mushroom frittata (using chickpea flour)

**Ingredients:**
- 1 cup chickpea flour
- 1 cup unsweetened almond milk
- 3 eggs
- 1 tbsp olive oil
- 8 oz cremini mushrooms, sliced
- 1 shallot, minced
- 3 cups fresh spinach, chopped
- 1/2 cup shredded vegan mozzarella cheese
- 1 tsp dried thyme
- Salt and pepper to taste

**Instructions:**

1. Preheat oven to 375°F. Grease a 9-inch pie dish or oven-safe skillet.

2. In a medium bowl, whisk together the chickpea flour and almond milk until smooth. Then whisk in the 3 eggs.

3. In a skillet, heat the olive oil over medium heat. Add the sliced mushrooms and minced shallot. Sauté for 5-7 minutes until the mushrooms are tender.

4. Add the chopped spinach to the skillet and cook for 2-3 minutes, until the spinach is wilted.

5. Pour the chickpea flour-egg mixture over the mushroom-spinach mixture in the skillet. Sprinkle the shredded vegan mozzarella and dried thyme on top.

6. Transfer the skillet to the preheated oven. Bake for 25-30 minutes, until the center is set and the top is lightly golden.

7. Let the frittata cool for 5-10 minutes before slicing and serving.

8. Season with salt and pepper to taste.

**This chickpea flour-based frittata is a delicious, protein-packed vegetarian breakfast or brunch dish. The spinach and mushrooms add great flavor and texture.**

# 25. Vegetable pad Thai

**Ingredients**:
- 8 oz rice noodles
- 2 tbsp tamarind paste
- 2 tbsp fish sauce (or soy sauce for vegan)
- 1 tbsp brown sugar
- 1 tbsp lime juice
- 2 tbsp vegetable oil
- 3 cloves garlic, minced
- 1 red bell pepper, thinly sliced
- 1 cup bean sprouts
- 1/2 cup shredded carrots
- 2 eggs, lightly beaten (or 2 tbsp chickpea flour for vegan)
- 2 green onions, sliced
- 1/4 cup chopped roasted peanuts
- Lime wedges for serving

**Instructions**:

1. Soak the rice noodles in hot water for 15-20 minutes until softened. Drain and set aside.

2. In a small bowl, whisk together the tamarind paste, fish sauce (or soy sauce), brown sugar, and lime juice. Set the sauce aside.

3. Heat the vegetable oil in a large skillet or wok over medium-high heat. Add the minced garlic and sauté for 1 minute until fragrant.

4. Add the sliced bell pepper, bean sprouts, and shredded carrots. Stir-fry for 3-4 minutes until vegetables are tender-crisp.

5. Push the vegetables to the side of the pan. Pour the beaten eggs (or chickpea flour mixed with 2 tbsp water for vegan) into the empty space and let cook for 30 seconds to 1 minute, then scramble.

6. Add the soaked rice noodles and the prepared sauce to the pan. Toss everything together for 2-3 minutes until the noodles are heated through and coated in the sauce.

7. Remove from heat and stir in the sliced green onions.

8. Serve the vegetable pad thai immediately, garnished with chopped roasted peanuts and lime wedges.

**This veggie-packed pad thai is a delicious meatless version of the classic Thai dish. Adjust the spice level to your preference.**

# 26. Lentil and vegetable soup

**Ingredients:**
- 1 cup dry brown or green lentils, rinsed
- 6 cups vegetable or chicken broth
- 2 tbsp olive oil
- 1 onion, diced
- 3 carrots, peeled and diced
- 3 celery stalks, diced
- 3 cloves garlic, minced
- 1 tsp dried thyme
- 1 tsp dried oregano
- 1 (15 oz) can diced tomatoes
- 2 cups chopped kale or spinach
- Salt and pepper to taste
- Chopped parsley for garnish

**Instructions:**

1. In a large pot, combine the rinsed lentils and broth. Bring to a boil over high heat.

2. Reduce heat to medium-low, cover and simmer the lentils for 15-20 minutes, until tender.

3. In a separate large pot or Dutch oven, heat the olive oil over medium heat. Add the diced onion, carrots, and celery. Sauté for 5-7 minutes until starting to soften.

4. Stir in the minced garlic, dried thyme, and dried oregano. Cook for 1 minute more.

5. Pour the cooked lentils and their broth into the pot with the sautéed vegetables.

6. Add the diced tomatoes and chopped kale or spinach. Season with salt and pepper.

7. Bring the soup to a simmer and cook for 10-15 minutes, until the vegetables are tender.

8. Ladle the lentil and vegetable soup into bowls and garnish with chopped fresh parsley.

*This hearty, nutritious soup is packed with protein from the lentils and fiber from the vegetables. It makes a satisfying meatless meal.*

# 27. Stuffed bell peppers with lentils and rice

**Ingredients:**
- 6 bell peppers, tops removed and seeds/membranes scooped out
- 1 cup cooked brown rice
- 1 cup cooked brown or green lentils
- 1 onion, diced
- 3 cloves garlic, minced
- 1 tsp dried oregano
- 1 tsp ground cumin
- 1/4 tsp cayenne pepper (optional)
- 1 (15 oz) can diced tomatoes
- 1/2 cup shredded cheddar or vegan cheese
- Salt and pepper to taste
- Chopped parsley for garnish

**Instructions:**
1. Preheat oven to 375°F. Arrange the hollowed-out bell peppers in a baking dish.

2. In a large skillet, sauté the diced onion in a bit of olive oil over medium heat for 5 minutes until translucent.

3. Add the minced garlic and cook for 1 minute more.

4. Stir in the cooked rice, cooked lentils, oregano, cumin, and cayenne (if using).

5. Pour in the diced tomatoes and their juices. Season with salt and pepper.

6. Spoon the lentil-rice filling into the hollowed bell peppers, packing it in tightly.

7. Top the stuffed peppers with the shredded cheese.

8. Cover the baking dish with foil and bake for 30 minutes.

9. Remove the foil and bake for 10-15 minutes more, until the peppers are tender and the cheese is melted.

10. Garnish the stuffed peppers with chopped fresh parsley before serving.

**These hearty, protein-packed stuffed bell peppers make a delicious vegetarian main dish. The lentil and rice filling is so flavorful.**

# 28. Tofu and vegetable stir-fry noodles

**Ingredients:**
- 8 oz rice noodles
- 1 block (14 oz) extra-firm tofu, pressed and cubed
- 2 tbsp sesame oil, divided
- 2 cups mixed vegetables (broccoli florets, sliced carrots, snow peas, etc.)
- 3 cloves garlic, minced
- 1 tbsp grated fresh ginger
- 2 tbsp low-sodium soy sauce
- 1 tbsp rice vinegar
- 1 tsp sesame oil
- Salt and pepper to taste
- Chopped green onions and toasted sesame seeds for garnish

**Instructions:**

1. Prepare the rice noodles according to package instructions. Drain and set aside.

2. In a large skillet or wok, heat 1 tbsp of the sesame oil over medium-high heat. Add the cubed tofu and cook for 5-7 minutes, turning occasionally, until lightly browned on all sides. Transfer tofu to a plate.

3. In the same pan, heat the remaining 1 tbsp sesame oil. Add the mixed vegetables and stir-fry for 3-4 minutes until starting to soften.

4. Push the vegetables to the side of the pan. Add the minced garlic and grated ginger to the empty space and cook for 1 minute until fragrant.

5. Add the cooked rice noodles, soy sauce, rice vinegar, and 1 tsp sesame oil to the pan. Toss everything together for 2-3 minutes until the noodles are heated through.

6. Gently fold the cooked tofu back into the stir-fry.

7. Season with salt and pepper to taste.

8. Serve the tofu and vegetable stir-fry noodles immediately, garnished with chopped green onions and toasted sesame seeds.

***This colorful, veggie-packed stir-fry makes a delicious meatless main dish. The tofu adds protein while the noodles make it a hearty meal.***

# 29. Mushroom and spinach stuffed shells

**Ingredients:**
- 12 oz jumbo pasta shells
- 2 tbsp olive oil
- 8 oz cremini mushrooms, finely chopped
- 1 onion, diced
- 3 cloves garlic, minced
- 5 oz fresh spinach, chopped
- 1 cup ricotta cheese
- 1/2 cup shredded mozzarella cheese
- 1/4 cup grated Parmesan cheese
- 1 egg
- 1 tsp dried oregano
- Salt and pepper to taste
- 1 (24 oz) jar marinara sauce

**Instructions:**

1. Preheat oven to 375°F. Cook the pasta shells according to package instructions until al dente. Drain and set aside.

2. In a skillet, heat the olive oil over medium heat. Add the chopped mushrooms and diced onion. Sauté for 5-7 minutes until the mushrooms are tender.

3. Stir in the minced garlic and chopped spinach. Cook for 2-3 minutes until the spinach is wilted. Remove from heat and let cool slightly.

4. In a medium bowl, mix together the sautéed mushroom-spinach mixture, ricotta cheese, mozzarella, Parmesan, egg, and dried oregano. Season with salt and pepper.

5. Spread 1 cup of the marinara sauce in the bottom of a 9x13 baking dish.

6. Stuff each cooked pasta shell with a spoonful of the mushroom-spinach filling. Arrange the stuffed shells in the baking dish.

7. Pour the remaining marinara sauce over the top of the stuffed shells.

8. Cover the dish with foil and bake for 25-30 minutes, until heated through.

9. Remove the foil and bake for 5 minutes more to lightly brown the tops.

10. Serve the mushroom and spinach stuffed shells warm. Enjoy!

# 30. Vegetarian pad Thai

**Ingredients:**
- 8 oz rice noodles
- 3 tbsp tamarind paste
- 2 tbsp soy sauce
- 1 tbsp brown sugar
- 1 tbsp lime juice
- 2 tbsp vegetable oil
- 3 cloves garlic, minced
- 1 cup diced firm tofu
- 1 cup shredded carrots
- 1 cup bean sprouts
- 2 eggs, lightly beaten (or 2 tbsp chickpea flour for vegan)
- 2 green onions, sliced
- 1/4 cup chopped roasted peanuts
- Lime wedges for serving

**Instructions:**

1. Soak the rice noodles in hot water for 15-20 minutes until softened. Drain and set aside.

2. In a small bowl, whisk together the tamarind paste, soy sauce, brown sugar, and lime juice. Set the sauce aside.

3. Heat the vegetable oil in a large skillet or wok over medium-high heat. Add the minced garlic and sauté for 1 minute until fragrant.

4. Add the diced tofu, shredded carrots, and bean sprouts. Stir-fry for 3-4 minutes until the vegetables are tender-crisp.

5. Push the tofu and vegetables to the side of the pan. Pour the beaten eggs (or chickpea flour mixed with 2 tbsp water for vegan) into the empty space and let cook for 30 seconds to 1 minute, then scramble.

6. Add the soaked rice noodles and the prepared sauce to the pan. Toss everything together for 2-3 minutes until the noodles are heated through and coated in the sauce.

7. Remove from heat and stir in the sliced green onions.

8. Serve the vegetarian pad thai immediately, garnished with chopped roasted peanuts and lime wedges.

*This meatless pad thai is packed with protein from the tofu and is a delicious vegetarian version of the classic Thai dish. Adjust the spice level to your preference.*

# 31. Quinoa stuffed eggplant

**Ingredients:**
- 2 medium eggplants, halved lengthwise
- 1 cup cooked quinoa
- 1 cup diced tomatoes
- 1/2 cup crumbled feta cheese
- 1/4 cup chopped fresh basil
- 2 cloves garlic, minced
- 1 tbsp olive oil
- Salt and pepper to taste

**Instructions:**

1. Preheat oven to 400°F. Scoop out the flesh from the eggplant halves, leaving about 1/4 inch of flesh attached to the skin. Chop the scooped out eggplant flesh.

2. In a bowl, combine the chopped eggplant flesh, quinoa, tomatoes, feta, basil, garlic, and olive oil. Season with salt and pepper.

3. Stuff the eggplant halves evenly with the quinoa mixture.

4. Place the stuffed eggplant halves on a baking sheet. Bake for 25-30 minutes, until the eggplant is tender and the filling is hot.

5. Serve warm. Enjoy!

# 32. Vegetable korma

**Ingredients:**
- 1 cup mixed vegetables (such as cauliflower, potatoes, carrots, peas)
- 1 onion, diced
- 3 cloves garlic, minced
- 1 inch ginger, grated
- 1 tsp cumin seeds
- 1 tsp coriander powder
- 1 tsp garam masala
- 1 tsp turmeric powder
- 1 tsp red chili powder (or to taste)
- 1 cup coconut milk
- 1 tbsp tomato paste
- Salt to taste
- Chopped cilantro for garnish

**Instructions:**

1. Heat oil in a pan. Add the cumin seeds and let them sizzle for a few seconds.

2. Add the diced onions and sauté until translucent. Then add the garlic and ginger and sauté for 1 minute.

3. Add the mixed vegetables and sauté for 2-3 minutes.

4. Add the coriander powder, garam masala, turmeric, and red chili powder. Stir to coat the vegetables.

5. Pour in the coconut milk and tomato paste. Stir well and bring to a simmer.

6. Cover and cook for 15-20 minutes, until the vegetables are tender.

7. Season with salt to taste.

8. Garnish with chopped cilantro and serve hot with naan or rice.

# 33. Tofu and vegetable curry

**Ingredients:**
- 1 block firm or extra-firm tofu, cubed
- 2 tbsp oil
- 1 onion, diced
- 3 cloves garlic, minced
- 1 inch ginger, grated
- 1 tsp cumin seeds
- 1 tsp coriander powder
- 1 tsp garam masala
- 1 tsp turmeric powder
- 1 tsp red chili powder (or to taste)
- 1 cup mixed vegetables (such as bell peppers, cauliflower, potatoes)
- 1 cup coconut milk
- 1 tbsp tomato paste
- Salt to taste
- Chopped cilantro for garnish

**Instructions**:

1. Heat oil in a pan. Add the cubed tofu and fry until golden brown on all sides. Remove and set aside.

2. In the same pan, add the cumin seeds and let them sizzle for a few seconds.

3. Add the diced onions and sauté until translucent. Then add the garlic and ginger and sauté for 1 minute.

4. Add the mixed vegetables and sauté for 2-3 minutes.

5. Add the coriander powder, garam masala, turmeric, and red chili powder. Stir to coat the vegetables.

6. Pour in the coconut milk and tomato paste. Stir well and bring to a simmer.

7. Add the fried tofu cubes and gently stir to combine.

8. Cover and cook for 15-20 minutes, until the vegetables are tender.

9. Season with salt to taste.

10. Garnish with chopped cilantro and serve hot with rice or naan.

# 34. Lentil moussaka

**Ingredients**:
***For the Lentil Filling:***
- 1 cup brown or green lentils, rinsed
- 1 onion, diced
- 3 cloves garlic, minced
- 1 tsp ground cinnamon
- 1 tsp dried oregano
- 1 tsp tomato paste
- 1 (14oz) can diced tomatoes
- Salt and pepper to taste

For the Eggplant Layers:
- 2 medium eggplants, sliced into 1/4 inch rounds
- 2 tbsp olive oil
- Salt and pepper to taste

***For the Béchamel Sauce:***
- 3 tbsp butter
- 3 tbsp all-purpose flour
- 2 cups milk
- 1/4 tsp ground nutmeg
- Salt and pepper to taste
- 1/2 cup grated Parmesan cheese

**Instructions:**
1. Preheat oven to 375°F.

2. Make the Lentil Filling: In a saucepan, cover the lentils with water and bring to a boil. Reduce heat and simmer for 15-20 minutes until tender. Drain and set aside.

3. In a skillet, sauté the onion and garlic until softened. Add the cooked lentils, cinnamon, oregano, tomato paste, and diced tomatoes. Season with salt and pepper. Simmer for 10 minutes.

4. Make the Eggplant Layers: Arrange the eggplant slices on baking sheets, brush with olive oil, and season with salt and pepper. Bake for 15-20 minutes until softened.

5. Make the Béchamel Sauce: In a saucepan, melt the butter over medium heat. Whisk in the flour and cook for 2 minutes. Gradually whisk in the milk and cook until thickened, about 5-7 minutes. Season with nutmeg, salt, and pepper.

6. Assemble the Moussaka: Spread half the lentil filling in the bottom of a 9x13 inch baking dish. Top with a layer of eggplant slices. Spread the béchamel sauce over the eggplant and sprinkle with Parmesan cheese. Repeat the layers.

7. Bake for 30-40 minutes, until the top is golden brown. Let stand for 10 minutes before serving.

# 35. Tofu and vegetable stir-fry with ginger soy sauce

**Ingredients:**
- 1 block firm or extra-firm tofu, cubed
- 2 tbsp vegetable oil
- 2 cups mixed vegetables (such as broccoli, bell peppers, snow peas, carrots)
- 3 cloves garlic, minced
- 1 inch ginger, grated

*For the Ginger Soy Sauce:*
- 3 tbsp soy sauce
- 2 tbsp rice vinegar
- 1 tbsp honey
- 1 tsp sesame oil
- 1 tsp grated ginger
- 1 tsp cornstarch

**Instructions**:

1. In a small bowl, whisk together all the ingredients for the ginger soy sauce. Set aside.

2. Heat the vegetable oil in a large skillet or wok over high heat.

3. Add the cubed tofu and stir-fry for 3-4 minutes until lightly browned on all sides. Remove the tofu from the pan and set aside.

4. Add the mixed vegetables to the hot pan and stir-fry for 3-4 minutes until crisp-tender.

5. Add the minced garlic and grated ginger to the pan and stir-fry for 1 minute until fragrant.

6. Pour the ginger soy sauce into the pan and bring to a simmer. Cook for 1-2 minutes until the sauce has thickened slightly.

7. Add the sautéed tofu back to the pan and gently toss everything together to coat the tofu and vegetables in the sauce.

8. Serve the tofu and vegetable stir-fry immediately, over steamed rice or noodles if desired. Enjoy!

# 36. Stuffed portobello mushrooms with quinoa and vegetables

**Ingredients:**
- 4 large portobello mushroom caps, stems removed and chopped
- 1 cup cooked quinoa
- 1 cup diced bell peppers
- 1/2 cup diced onion
- 2 cloves garlic, minced
- 1/2 cup diced tomatoes
- 1/4 cup crumbled feta cheese
- 2 tbsp chopped fresh basil
- 1 tbsp olive oil
- Salt and pepper to taste

**Instructions**:

1. Preheat oven to 400°F. Lightly grease a baking sheet.

2. Place the portobello mushroom caps, gill-side up, on the prepared baking sheet. Bake for 10 minutes to partially cook.

3. In a skillet, heat the olive oil over medium heat. Add the chopped mushroom stems, bell peppers, onion, and garlic. Sauté for 5-7 minutes until vegetables are tender.

4. Remove the skillet from heat and stir in the cooked quinoa, diced tomatoes, feta cheese, and fresh basil. Season with salt and pepper.

5. Spoon the quinoa and vegetable mixture evenly into the baked portobello caps.

6. Return the stuffed mushrooms to the oven and bake for an additional 15-20 minutes, until the mushrooms are tender and the filling is hot.

7. Serve the stuffed portobello mushrooms warm. Enjoy!

***You can customize the vegetables used in the filling based on your preferences. Some other options include spinach, zucchini, or artichoke hearts.***

# 37. Chickpea and vegetable tagine

**Ingredients:**
- 1 tbsp olive oil
- 1 onion, diced
- 3 cloves garlic, minced
- 1 tsp ground cumin
- 1 tsp ground coriander
- 1 tsp paprika
- 1/2 tsp ground cinnamon
- 1/4 tsp cayenne pepper (or to taste)
- 1 (15oz) can chickpeas, drained and rinsed
- 1 (14oz) can diced tomatoes
- 2 cups vegetable broth
- 2 medium carrots, peeled and sliced
- 1 medium zucchini, sliced
- 1 cup cauliflower florets
- Salt and pepper to taste
- Chopped cilantro for garnish

**Instructions:**

1. Heat the olive oil in a large pot or tagine over medium heat. Add the diced onion and sauté for 5 minutes until translucent.

2. Add the minced garlic and spices (cumin, coriander, paprika, cinnamon, cayenne). Stir and cook for 1 minute until fragrant.

3. Stir in the chickpeas, diced tomatoes, and vegetable broth. Bring the mixture to a simmer.

4. Add the sliced carrots, zucchini, and cauliflower florets. Season with salt and pepper.

5. Cover and simmer for 20-25 minutes, until the vegetables are tender.

6. Taste and adjust seasoning as needed.

7. Serve the chickpea and vegetable tagine warm, garnished with chopped cilantro. Can be served over couscous or with crusty bread.

This tagine is full of flavor from the aromatic spices and makes a hearty, vegetable-packed meal.

# 38. Stuffed sweet potatoes with black beans and corn

**Ingredients:**
- 4 medium sweet potatoes
- 1 (15oz) can black beans, drained and rinsed
- 1 cup frozen corn kernels
- 1/2 cup salsa
- 1 tsp chili powder
- 1/2 tsp cumin
- 1/4 tsp garlic powder
- Salt and pepper to taste
- 1/2 cup shredded cheddar or monterey jack cheese
- Chopped cilantro for garnish

**Instructions:**

1. Preheat oven to 400°F. Pierce the sweet potatoes several times with a fork and place them directly on the oven rack. Bake for 45-60 minutes, until very soft when squeezed.

2. Remove the sweet potatoes from the oven and let cool slightly. Cut each potato in half lengthwise.

3. Scoop out the flesh from the sweet potato halves, leaving about 1/4 inch of flesh attached to the skin. Place the scooped out flesh in a bowl.

4. To the bowl with the sweet potato flesh, add the black beans, corn, salsa, chili powder, cumin, garlic powder, and a pinch of salt and pepper. Mash and stir to combine.

5. Spoon the black bean and corn mixture back into the sweet potato skins, dividing it evenly.

6. Top each stuffed sweet potato half with shredded cheese.

7. Return the stuffed sweet potatoes to the oven and bake for an additional 10-15 minutes, until the cheese is melted.

8. Garnish the stuffed sweet potatoes with chopped cilantro before serving.

# 39. Vegan sushi rolls with avocado and cucumber

**Ingredients:**
- 1 cup short-grain sushi rice
- 2 tbsp rice vinegar
- 1 tsp sugar
- 1/2 tsp salt
- 1 avocado, sliced
- 1 cucumber, peeled and cut into thin strips
- 4-6 sheets of nori (seaweed sheets)
- Soy sauce, for serving
- Wasabi, for serving (optional)

**Instructions**:

1. Cook the sushi rice according to package instructions. Transfer to a large bowl and let cool slightly.

2. In a small bowl, mix together the rice vinegar, sugar, and salt. Pour this mixture over the cooked rice and gently fold to combine. Allow the rice to cool completely.

3. Lay a sheet of nori on a bamboo sushi mat or clean surface. Spread about 1/2 cup of the seasoned sushi rice evenly over the nori, leaving about 1 inch of nori uncovered at the top.

4. Arrange a few slices of avocado and cucumber strips in a line across the center of the rice.

5. Carefully lift the edge of the sushi mat closest to you and roll the nori tightly over the filling, using the mat to guide the roll. Continue rolling until you reach the uncovered edge of the nori, then moisten with water to seal the roll.

6. Repeat with the remaining nori sheets and fillings to make 4-6 sushi rolls.

7. Using a sharp knife, slice each roll into 6-8 pieces.

8. Serve the vegan sushi rolls with soy sauce and wasabi on the side, if desired.

# 40. Lentil and vegetable biryani

**Ingredients:**
- 1 cup brown or green lentils, rinsed
- 2 cups basmati rice
- 3 tbsp oil
- 1 onion, diced
- 3 cloves garlic, minced
- 1 inch ginger, grated
- 1 tsp cumin seeds
- 1 tsp coriander powder
- 1 tsp garam masala
- 1 tsp turmeric powder
- 1 tsp red chili powder (or to taste)
- 2 cups mixed vegetables (such as cauliflower, carrots, peas)
- 1 cup diced tomatoes
- 1 cup water or vegetable broth
- Salt to taste
- Chopped cilantro for garnish

**Instructions:**
1. Cook the lentils: In a saucepan, cover the lentils with water and bring to a boil. Reduce heat and simmer for 15-20 minutes until tender. Drain and set aside.

2. Cook the rice: In a separate pot, cook the basmati rice according to package instructions. Fluff with a fork and set aside.

3. In a large skillet or pot, heat the oil over medium heat. Add the cumin seeds and let them sizzle for a few seconds.

4. Add the diced onion and sauté until translucent. Then add the garlic and ginger and sauté for 1 minute.

5. Add the coriander powder, garam masala, turmeric, and red chili powder. Stir to coat the onions.

6. Add the mixed vegetables and sauté for 2-3 minutes.

7. Stir in the cooked lentils, diced tomatoes, and water/broth. Season with salt.

8. Bring the mixture to a simmer, then reduce heat and let it cook for 15-20 minutes, until the vegetables are tender.

9. Gently fold the cooked rice into the lentil-vegetable mixture until well combined. Garnish with chopped cilantro and serve hot.

# 41. Vegetable curry with tofu

**Ingredients:**
- 1 block firm or extra-firm tofu, cubed
- 2 tbsp oil
- 1 onion, diced
- 3 cloves garlic, minced
- 1 inch ginger, grated
- 1 tsp cumin seeds
- 1 tsp coriander powder
- 1 tsp garam masala
- 1 tsp turmeric powder
- 1 tsp red chili powder (or to taste)
- 2 cups mixed vegetables (such as cauliflower, potatoes, carrots, peas)
- 1 cup coconut milk
- 1 tbsp tomato paste
- Salt to taste
- Chopped cilantro for garnish

**Instructions:**

1. Heat oil in a pan. Add the cubed tofu and fry until golden brown on all sides. Remove and set aside.

2. In the same pan, add the cumin seeds and let them sizzle for a few seconds.

3. Add the diced onion and sauté until translucent. Then add the garlic and ginger and sauté for 1 minute.

4. Add the mixed vegetables and sauté for 2-3 minutes.

5. Add the coriander powder, garam masala, turmeric, and red chili powder. Stir to coat the vegetables.

6. Pour in the coconut milk and tomato paste. Stir well and bring to a simmer. Add the fried tofu cubes and gently stir to combine.

7. Cover and cook for 15-20 minutes, until the vegetables are tender. Season with salt to taste. Garnish with chopped cilantro and serve hot with rice or naan.

**This vegetable curry with tofu is a delicious and nutritious meatless main dish. The combination of spices, coconut milk, and vegetables creates a flavorful and creamy curry. Let me know if you have any other questions!**

# 42. Stuffed bell peppers with quinoa and black beans

**Ingredients:**
- 4 large bell peppers, halved lengthwise and seeds/membranes removed
- 1 cup cooked quinoa
- 1 (15oz) can black beans, drained and rinsed
- 1 cup diced tomatoes
- 1/2 cup diced onion
- 2 cloves garlic, minced
- 1 tsp chili powder
- 1 tsp cumin
- 1/4 tsp cayenne pepper (optional)
- Salt and pepper to taste
- 1/2 cup shredded cheddar or monterey jack cheese

**Instructions:**

1. Preheat oven to 375°F. Arrange the bell pepper halves in a baking dish.

2. In a bowl, combine the cooked quinoa, black beans, diced tomatoes, onion, garlic, chili powder, cumin, cayenne (if using), and season with salt and pepper.

3. Spoon the quinoa and black bean mixture evenly into the bell pepper halves.

4. Top each stuffed pepper with the shredded cheese.

5. Cover the baking dish with foil and bake for 30 minutes.

6. Remove the foil and bake for an additional 10-15 minutes, until the peppers are tender and the cheese is melted.

7. Serve the stuffed bell peppers warm. Garnish with chopped cilantro or green onions if desired.

*These stuffed bell peppers are a delicious and nutritious vegetarian main dish. The quinoa and black beans provide protein, while the bell peppers add a nice crunch and sweetness. Feel free to adjust the spices to your taste. Enjoy!*

# 43. Tofu and vegetable bibimbap bowl

**Ingredients:**
***For the Tofu:***
- 1 block firm or extra-firm tofu, cubed
- 1 tbsp soy sauce
- 1 tsp sesame oil
- 1 tsp rice vinegar
- 1 tsp brown sugar

***For the Vegetables:***
- 2 cups mixed vegetables (such as spinach, carrots, bean sprouts, mushrooms)
- 1 tbsp sesame oil
- 1 tbsp soy sauce
- 1 tsp rice vinegar

***For the Bibimbap Bowl:***
- 2 cups cooked short-grain rice
- 2 eggs, fried or cooked sunny-side up
- 1 tbsp sesame seeds
- Gochujang (Korean chili paste), for serving

**Instructions:**
1. Make the Tofu: In a bowl, combine the cubed tofu, soy sauce, sesame oil, rice vinegar, and brown sugar. Toss to coat. Heat a skillet over medium-high heat and sauté the tofu until browned on all sides, about 5-7 minutes. Set aside.

2. Make the Vegetables: In the same skillet, heat the sesame oil over medium heat. Add the mixed vegetables and sauté for 3-5 minutes until tender. Stir in the soy sauce and rice vinegar. Remove from heat.

3. Assemble the Bibimbap Bowl: Divide the cooked rice between two bowls. Top each bowl with the sautéed tofu, vegetables, and a fried or sunny-side up egg.

4. Sprinkle the bibimbap bowls with sesame seeds.

5. Serve the bibimbap with gochujang (Korean chili paste) on the side, allowing each person to add as much or as little as they like.

Stir everything together before eating to combine all the flavors. The runny egg yolk helps bind the rice, tofu, and vegetables together.

# 44. Lentil and vegetable birria tacos

**Ingredients:**
*For the Lentil Birria:*
- 1 cup brown or green lentils, rinsed
- 1 onion, diced
- 3 cloves garlic, minced
- 1 tbsp chili powder
- 1 tsp cumin
- 1 tsp oregano
- 1 tsp smoked paprika
- 1 (14oz) can diced tomatoes
- 2 cups vegetable broth
- Salt and pepper to taste

*For the Tacos:*
- 12-16 corn tortillas
- 1 cup shredded mozzarella or Oaxaca cheese
- Chopped onion, cilantro, and lime wedges for serving

**Instructions:**
1. Make the Lentil Birria: In a large pot, combine the lentils, onion, garlic, chili powder, cumin, oregano, and smoked paprika. Pour in the diced tomatoes and vegetable broth. Season with salt and pepper.

2. Bring the mixture to a boil, then reduce heat and simmer for 20-25 minutes, until the lentils are very tender. Use a potato masher or the back of a spoon to slightly mash some of the lentils to thicken the stew.

3. Preheat oven to 400°F. Wrap the corn tortillas in foil and warm in the oven for 5-10 minutes.

4. To assemble the tacos, place a spoonful of the lentil birria in the center of each warm tortilla. Top with shredded cheese, chopped onion, and cilantro.

5. Serve the lentil birria tacos immediately, with lime wedges on the side for squeezing over the top.

The lentil birria filling can also be used to make quesadillas, burritos, or served over rice. The smoky, spiced lentils make a delicious vegetarian alternative to traditional beef birria.

# 45. Quinoa stuffed bell peppers

**Ingredients:**
- 4 large bell peppers, halved lengthwise and seeds/membranes removed
- 1 cup cooked quinoa
- 1 (15oz) can black beans, drained and rinsed
- 1 cup diced tomatoes
- 1/2 cup diced onion
- 2 cloves garlic, minced
- 1 tsp chili powder
- 1 tsp cumin
- 1/4 tsp cayenne pepper (optional)
- Salt and pepper to taste
- 1/2 cup shredded cheddar or monterey jack cheese

**Instructions**:

1. Preheat oven to 375°F. Arrange the bell pepper halves in a baking dish.

2. In a bowl, combine the cooked quinoa, black beans, diced tomatoes, onion, garlic, chili powder, cumin, cayenne (if using), and season with salt and pepper.

3. Spoon the quinoa and black bean mixture evenly into the bell pepper halves.

4. Top each stuffed pepper with the shredded cheese.

5. Cover the baking dish with foil and bake for 30 minutes.

6. Remove the foil and bake for an additional 10-15 minutes, until the peppers are tender and the cheese is melted.

7. Serve the stuffed bell peppers warm. Garnish with chopped cilantro or green onions if desired.

***These quinoa stuffed bell peppers are a delicious and nutritious vegetarian main dish. The quinoa and black beans provide protein, while the bell peppers add a nice crunch and sweetness. Feel free to adjust the spices to your taste. Enjoy!***

# 46. Tofu and vegetable pho

**Ingredients:**
- 8 cups vegetable broth
- 3 whole star anise
- 3 whole cloves
- 1 cinnamon stick
- 1 tablespoon grated fresh ginger
- 1 tablespoon soy sauce
- 1 teaspoon brown sugar
- 8 oz firm or extra-firm tofu, cubed
- 8 oz rice noodles
- 2 cups thinly sliced mixed vegetables (such as carrots, cabbage, bean sprouts, mushrooms)
- 1/4 cup chopped fresh cilantro
- 2 green onions, thinly sliced
- Lime wedges for serving

**Instructions**:
1. In a large pot, combine the vegetable broth, star anise, cloves, cinnamon stick, ginger, soy sauce, and brown sugar. Bring to a boil over high heat.

2. Reduce heat to medium-low and let the broth simmer for 15-20 minutes to allow the flavors to infuse.

3. Add the tofu cubes and rice noodles to the simmering broth. Cook for 5-7 minutes until the noodles are tender.

4. Stir in the sliced vegetables and cook for 2-3 minutes more, until the vegetables are crisp-tender.

5. Remove the star anise, cloves, and cinnamon stick from the broth.

6. Ladle the pho into bowls and top with the chopped cilantro and green onions.

7. Serve immediately with lime wedges on the side.

# 47. Stuffed acorn squash with wild rice and cranberries

**Ingredients:**
- 2 acorn squash, halved and seeded
- 1 cup cooked wild rice
- 1/2 cup dried cranberries
- 1/4 cup chopped pecans
- 2 tablespoons maple syrup
- 1 teaspoon ground cinnamon
- 1/4 teaspoon ground nutmeg
- Salt and pepper to taste
- 2 tablespoons olive oil

**Instructions**:
1. Preheat your oven to 400°F (200°C).

2. Place the acorn squash halves cut-side up on a baking sheet. Brush the insides with olive oil and season with salt and pepper.

3. Bake the squash for 30-40 minutes, or until tender when pierced with a fork.

4. In a medium bowl, combine the cooked wild rice, dried cranberries, chopped pecans, maple syrup, cinnamon, and nutmeg. Season with salt and pepper to taste.

5. Scoop the wild rice mixture into the baked acorn squash halves, dividing it evenly.

6. Return the stuffed squash to the oven and bake for an additional 15-20 minutes, or until the filling is heated through and the squash is very tender.

7. Serve the stuffed acorn squash warm, garnished with extra pecans or cranberries if desired.

***Enjoy this delicious and festive stuffed acorn squash dish! The combination of the sweet and nutty wild rice, tart cranberries, and warm spices is simply delightful.***

# 48. Vegetable and tofu stir-fry with peanut sauce

**Ingredients**:
- 1 block (14 oz) firm or extra-firm tofu, cubed
- 2 tablespoons vegetable oil
- 3 cloves garlic, minced
- 1 inch fresh ginger, grated
- 1 red bell pepper, sliced
- 1 cup broccoli florets
- 1 cup sliced mushrooms
- 1 cup snow peas or snap peas
- 2 green onions, sliced
- 1/4 cup creamy peanut butter
- 2 tablespoons soy sauce
- 1 tablespoon rice vinegar
- 1 tablespoon honey or maple syrup
- 1 teaspoon sesame oil
- 1/4 cup water or vegetable broth
- Salt and pepper to taste
- Chopped peanuts and cilantro for garnish (optional)

**Instructions:**

1. In a large skillet or wok, heat the vegetable oil over medium-high heat. Add the cubed tofu and cook, stirring occasionally, until lightly browned on all sides, about 5-7 minutes. Transfer the tofu to a plate.

2. In the same skillet, add the minced garlic and grated ginger. Cook for 1 minute, stirring constantly, until fragrant.

3. Add the sliced bell pepper, broccoli, mushrooms, and snow peas to the skillet. Stir-fry for 3-5 minutes, until the vegetables are crisp-tender.

4. In a small bowl, whisk together the peanut butter, soy sauce, rice vinegar, honey, sesame oil, and water or broth until well combined.

5. Add the cooked tofu and the peanut sauce to the skillet with the vegetables. Toss everything together and cook for 2-3 minutes, until the sauce has thickened and the tofu is heated through.

6. Remove from heat and stir in the sliced green onions. Season with salt and pepper to taste.

7. Serve the vegetable and tofu stir-fry over rice or noodles. Garnish with chopped peanuts and fresh cilantro, if desired.

# 49. Stuffed portobello mushrooms with spinach and quinoa

**Ingredients**:
- 4 large portobello mushroom caps, stems removed and chopped
- 1 cup cooked quinoa
- 1 cup fresh spinach, chopped
- 1/2 cup crumbled feta cheese
- 2 cloves garlic, minced
- 2 tablespoons olive oil
- 1 teaspoon dried oregano
- Salt and pepper to taste

**Instructions:**

1. Preheat your oven to 400°F (200°C).

2. Gently clean the portobello mushroom caps with a damp cloth. Remove the stems and chop them.

3. In a skillet, heat the olive oil over medium heat. Add the chopped mushroom stems, minced garlic, and sauté for 2-3 minutes until fragrant.

4. Add the chopped spinach to the skillet and cook for 1-2 minutes, until the spinach is wilted.

5. Transfer the spinach and mushroom mixture to a bowl. Add the cooked quinoa and crumbled feta cheese. Season with dried oregano, salt, and pepper. Mix well.

6. Arrange the portobello mushroom caps, gill-side up, on a baking sheet. Spoon the quinoa and spinach mixture evenly into the mushroom caps.

7. Bake the stuffed portobello mushrooms for 15-20 minutes, or until the mushrooms are tender and the filling is heated through.

8. Remove the stuffed mushrooms from the oven and let them cool for a few minutes before serving.

Serve the stuffed portobello mushrooms warm, garnished with extra feta cheese or fresh herbs if desired.

***Enjoy this delicious and healthy vegetarian dish! The combination of the earthy mushrooms, nutrient-rich quinoa, and fresh spinach makes for a satisfying and flavorful meal.***

# 50. Quinoa and vegetable bibimbap bowl

**Ingredients:**
- 1 cup uncooked quinoa, rinsed
- 2 cups vegetable broth
- 1 cup shredded carrots
- 1 cup thinly sliced zucchini
- 1 cup thinly sliced mushrooms
- 1 cup baby spinach leaves
- 2 eggs, fried or soft-boiled
- 2 tablespoons sesame seeds
- 2 tablespoons gochujang (Korean chili paste)
- 1 tablespoon sesame oil
- 1 tablespoon rice vinegar
- 1 teaspoon honey
- Salt and pepper to taste

**Instructions:**

1. Cook the quinoa: In a medium saucepan, combine the rinsed quinoa and vegetable broth. Bring to a boil, then reduce heat to low, cover, and simmer for 15-20 minutes, until the quinoa is tender and the liquid is absorbed. Fluff with a fork.

2. Prepare the vegetables: In a large skillet or wok, sauté the carrots, zucchini, and mushrooms over medium-high heat until tender-crisp, about 5-7 minutes. Add the spinach and cook for 1-2 minutes more, until wilted.

3. Make the bibimbap sauce: In a small bowl, whisk together the gochujang, sesame oil, rice vinegar, and honey. Season with salt and pepper to taste.

4. Assemble the bowls: Divide the cooked quinoa among 4 serving bowls. Top each bowl with the sautéed vegetables, a fried or soft-boiled egg, and a drizzle of the bibimbap sauce. Sprinkle with sesame seeds.

5. Serve immediately, allowing each person to mix the ingredients together in their bowl before eating.

*Enjoy this colorful and flavorful Quinoa and Vegetable Bibimbap Bowl! The combination of the nutty quinoa, fresh vegetables, and spicy-sweet bibimbap sauce makes for a delicious and nutritious meal.*

# 51. Chickpea and vegetable curry

**Ingredients**:
- 1 tablespoon olive oil
- 1 onion, diced
- 3 cloves garlic, minced
- 1 tablespoon grated fresh ginger
- 2 teaspoons garam masala
- 1 teaspoon ground cumin
- 1 teaspoon ground coriander
- 1/2 teaspoon ground turmeric
- 1/4 teaspoon cayenne pepper (or to taste)
- 1 (15 oz) can chickpeas, drained and rinsed
- 1 (14 oz) can diced tomatoes
- 1 cup vegetable broth
- 1 medium potato, peeled and diced
- 1 cup cauliflower florets
- 1 cup frozen peas
- 1 cup spinach leaves
- 1/4 cup chopped fresh cilantro
- Salt and pepper to taste
- Cooked basmati rice, for serving

**Instructions**:
1. In a large skillet or Dutch oven, heat the olive oil over medium heat. Add the diced onion and sauté for 5-7 minutes, until translucent.

2. Add the minced garlic and grated ginger to the skillet. Cook for 1 minute, until fragrant.

3. Stir in the garam masala, cumin, coriander, turmeric, and cayenne pepper. Cook for 2-3 minutes, stirring constantly, to toast the spices.

4. Add the drained and rinsed chickpeas, diced tomatoes, and vegetable broth. Bring the mixture to a simmer.

5. Add the diced potato, cauliflower florets, and frozen peas. Simmer for 15-20 minutes, until the vegetables are tender.

6. Stir in the spinach leaves and chopped cilantro. Cook for 2-3 minutes more, until the spinach is wilted.

7. Season the curry with salt and pepper to taste. Serve the chickpea and vegetable curry over cooked basmati rice. Garnish with additional cilantro if desired.

# 52. Lentil and vegetable pot pie

**Ingredients**:
*For the Filling:*
- 1 cup brown or green lentils, rinsed
- 4 cups vegetable broth
- 1 tablespoon olive oil
- 1 onion, diced
- 3 carrots, peeled and diced
- 2 celery stalks, diced
- 3 cloves garlic, minced
- 1 teaspoon dried thyme
- 1 teaspoon dried rosemary
- Salt and pepper to taste

*For the Crust:*
- 1 1/2 cups all-purpose flour
- 1/2 teaspoon salt
- 1/2 cup cold unsalted butter, cubed
- 1/4 cup ice water

**Instructions:**

*1. Make the Filling:*
   - In a medium saucepan, combine the lentils and vegetable broth. Bring to a boil, then reduce heat and simmer for 20-25 minutes, until the lentils are tender. Drain any excess liquid and set aside.
   - In a large skillet, heat the olive oil over medium heat. Add the diced onion, carrots, and celery. Sauté for 5-7 minutes, until the vegetables are softened.
   - Add the minced garlic, dried thyme, and dried rosemary. Cook for 1 minute, until fragrant.
   - Stir in the cooked lentils and season with salt and pepper to taste. Set the filling aside.

*2. Make the Crust:*
   - In a food processor, combine the flour and salt. Add the cold cubed butter and pulse until the mixture resembles coarse crumbs.
   - Add the ice water 1 tablespoon at a time, pulsing until the dough just begins to come together.
   - Turn the dough out onto a lightly floured surface and gently shape it into a disk. Wrap in plastic wrap and refrigerate for at least 30 minutes.

*3. Assemble and Bake the Pot Pie:*
   - Preheat your oven to 400°F (200°C).
   - Transfer the lentil and vegetable filling to a 9-inch pie dish or baking dish.
   - Roll out the chilled dough to a size that will fit over the top of the pie dish. Place the dough over the filling, pressing the edges to seal.
   - Cut a few slits in the top of the dough to allow steam to escape.
   - Bake the pot pie for 30-35 minutes, until the crust is golden brown and the filling is bubbling. Let the pot pie cool for 10-15 minutes before serving.

*Enjoy this hearty and comforting lentil and vegetable pot pie! The flaky crust and savory filling make for a delicious vegetarian main dish. Let me know if you have any other questions.*

# 53. Stuffed tomatoes with quinoa and spinach

**Ingredients:**
- 6 medium tomatoes
- 1 cup cooked quinoa
- 1 cup fresh spinach, chopped
- 1/2 cup crumbled feta cheese
- 2 tablespoons chopped fresh basil
- 2 cloves garlic, minced
- 1 tablespoon olive oil
- Salt and pepper to taste

**Instructions:**

1. Preheat your oven to 375°F (190°C).

2. Cut the tops off the tomatoes and scoop out the insides, reserving the pulp. Chop the tomato pulp.

3. In a medium bowl, combine the chopped tomato pulp, cooked quinoa, chopped spinach, crumbled feta cheese, chopped basil, and minced garlic. Mix well and season with salt and pepper to taste.

4. Stuff the tomato shells with the quinoa and spinach mixture, packing it in tightly.

5. Place the stuffed tomatoes in a baking dish. Drizzle the tops with the olive oil.

6. Bake the stuffed tomatoes for 20-25 minutes, or until the tomatoes are softened and the filling is heated through.

7. Serve the stuffed tomatoes warm, garnished with additional fresh basil if desired.

***Enjoy these delicious and nutritious Stuffed Tomatoes with Quinoa and Spinach! The combination of the juicy tomatoes, fluffy quinoa, and fresh spinach and herbs makes for a flavorful and satisfying vegetarian dish.***

# 54. Tofu and vegetable pad Thai

**Ingredients:**
- 8 oz rice noodles
- 2 tablespoons vegetable oil
- 1 block (14 oz) firm or extra-firm tofu, cubed
- 2 cloves garlic, minced
- 1 cup thinly sliced carrots
- 1 cup bean sprouts
- 1 cup chopped green cabbage
- 2 green onions, sliced
- 1/4 cup chopped roasted peanuts
- 2 tablespoons chopped fresh cilantro

*For the Sauce:*
- 3 tablespoons fish sauce (or soy sauce for a vegetarian/vegan version)
- 2 tablespoons lime juice
- 2 tablespoons brown sugar
- 1 tablespoon soy sauce
- 1 teaspoon Sriracha or other hot sauce (optional)

**Instructions:**
1. Soak the rice noodles in hot water for 15-20 minutes, until softened. Drain and set aside.

2. In a small bowl, whisk together all the sauce ingredients and set aside.

3. In a large skillet or wok, heat the vegetable oil over medium-high heat. Add the cubed tofu and cook, stirring occasionally, until lightly browned on all sides, about 5-7 minutes. Transfer the tofu to a plate.

4. In the same skillet, add the minced garlic and sauté for 1 minute until fragrant.

5. Add the sliced carrots, bean sprouts, and chopped cabbage to the skillet. Stir-fry for 3-5 minutes, until the vegetables are crisp-tender.

6. Add the cooked rice noodles and the prepared sauce to the skillet. Toss everything together until the noodles are well coated and heated through, about 2-3 minutes.

7. Stir in the cooked tofu and the sliced green onions. Cook for 1-2 minutes more.

8. Remove from heat and garnish the pad Thai with chopped roasted peanuts and fresh cilantro.

# 55. Stuffed mushrooms with quinoa and spinach

**Ingredients:**
- 12 large mushrooms, stems removed and chopped
- 1 cup cooked quinoa
- 1 cup fresh spinach, chopped
- 1/4 cup grated Parmesan cheese
- 2 cloves garlic, minced
- 2 tablespoons olive oil
- 1 teaspoon dried thyme
- Salt and pepper to taste

**Instructions**:

1. Preheat your oven to 375°F (190°C).

2. Clean the mushroom caps with a damp cloth and remove the stems. Finely chop the stems.

3. In a skillet, heat the olive oil over medium heat. Add the chopped mushroom stems and minced garlic. Sauté for 2-3 minutes until fragrant.

4. Add the chopped spinach to the skillet and cook for 1-2 minutes, until the spinach is wilted. Remove from heat and let cool slightly.

5. In a medium bowl, combine the sautéed mushroom stem and spinach mixture with the cooked quinoa and grated Parmesan cheese. Season with dried thyme, salt, and pepper.

6. Arrange the mushroom caps, gill-side up, on a baking sheet. Spoon the quinoa and spinach filling into the mushroom caps, dividing it evenly.

7. Bake the stuffed mushrooms for 15-20 minutes, or until the mushrooms are tender and the filling is heated through.

8. Remove the stuffed mushrooms from the oven and let them cool for a few minutes before serving.

Serve the Stuffed Mushrooms with Quinoa and Spinach warm, garnished with additional Parmesan cheese or fresh herbs if desired.

***Enjoy this delightful vegetarian appetizer or side dish! The combination of the earthy mushrooms, nutty quinoa, and fresh spinach makes for a flavorful and satisfying stuffed mushroom.***

# 56. Tofu and vegetable sushi bowl

**Ingredients:**
- 1 cup uncooked short-grain brown rice
- 2 cups water
- 1/4 cup rice vinegar
- 2 tablespoons sugar
- 1 teaspoon salt
- 1 block (14 oz) firm or extra-firm tofu, cubed
- 1 tablespoon sesame oil
- 1 carrot, julienned or shredded
- 1 cucumber, julienned or shredded
- 1 avocado, sliced
- 1 cup shredded purple cabbage
- 2 tablespoons toasted sesame seeds
- 2 tablespoons chopped fresh cilantro
- Soy sauce, for serving

**Instructions:**

1. Cook the brown rice: In a medium saucepan, combine the brown rice and water. Bring to a boil, then reduce heat to low, cover, and simmer for 25-30 minutes, until the rice is tender and the water is absorbed. Fluff with a fork.

2. Make the sushi rice: In a small bowl, whisk together the rice vinegar, sugar, and salt until the sugar has dissolved. Pour the vinegar mixture over the cooked brown rice and gently mix to combine. Set aside.

3. Cook the tofu: In a large skillet, heat the sesame oil over medium-high heat. Add the cubed tofu and cook, stirring occasionally, until lightly browned on all sides, about 5-7 minutes.

4. Assemble the sushi bowls: Divide the sushi rice among 4 serving bowls. Top each bowl with the cooked tofu, julienned carrots, julienned cucumber, sliced avocado, and shredded purple cabbage.

5. Sprinkle the sushi bowls with toasted sesame seeds and chopped fresh cilantro. Serve the Tofu and Vegetable Sushi Bowls with soy sauce on the side for drizzling or dipping.

*Enjoy this colorful and flavorful Tofu and Vegetable Sushi Bowl! The combination of the seasoned sushi rice, crisp vegetables, and savory tofu makes for a delicious and satisfying meal. Feel free to adjust the toppings to your liking.*

# 57. Lentil and vegetable birria tacos

**Ingredients:**
*For the Birria Filling:*
- 1 cup brown or green lentils, rinsed
- 4 cups vegetable broth
- 2 tablespoons olive oil
- 1 onion, diced
- 3 cloves garlic, minced
- 2 chipotle chiles in adobo sauce, minced
- 2 teaspoons chili powder
- 1 teaspoon ground cumin
- 1 teaspoon dried oregano
- 1 bay leaf
- Salt and pepper to taste

*For the Tacos:*
- 12-16 corn tortillas
- Shredded cabbage or lettuce
- Diced onion
- Chopped cilantro
- Lime wedges for serving
- Consommé (broth from the birria filling) for dipping

**Instructions:**

*1. Make the Birria Filling:*
- In a medium saucepan, combine the lentils and vegetable broth. Bring to a boil, then reduce heat and simmer for 20-25 minutes, until the lentils are tender. Drain any excess liquid and set aside.
- In a large skillet, heat the olive oil over medium heat. Add the diced onion and sauté for 5-7 minutes, until translucent.
- Add the minced garlic, chipotle chiles, chili powder, cumin, oregano, and bay leaf. Cook for 2-3 minutes, until fragrant.
- Stir in the cooked lentils and season with salt and pepper to taste. Simmer for 10 minutes, allowing the flavors to meld.

*2. Assemble the Tacos:*
- Warm the corn tortillas according to package instructions.
- Spoon the lentil birria filling into the center of each tortilla.
- Top with shredded cabbage or lettuce, diced onion, and chopped cilantro.
- Serve the tacos with lime wedges and the reserved consommé (broth) for dipping.

**Enjoy these delicious and flavorful Lentil and Vegetable Birria Tacos! The spicy, savory lentil filling paired with the fresh toppings and tangy consommé makes for a truly satisfying vegetarian taco experience.**

# 58. Quinoa stuffed bell peppers

**Ingredients:**
- 4 large bell peppers (any color)
- 1 cup cooked quinoa
- 1 (15 oz) can black beans, drained and rinsed
- 1 cup diced tomatoes (canned or fresh)
- 1/2 cup crumbled feta cheese
- 1/4 cup chopped fresh parsley
- 2 cloves garlic, minced
- 1 teaspoon ground cumin
- 1/2 teaspoon chili powder
- Salt and pepper to taste
- Shredded cheese (optional, for topping)

**Instructions**:

1. Preheat your oven to 375°F (190°C).

2. Cut the tops off the bell peppers and remove the seeds and membranes. Place the peppers in a baking dish.

3. In a medium bowl, combine the cooked quinoa, black beans, diced tomatoes, crumbled feta cheese, chopped parsley, minced garlic, cumin, chili powder, and salt and pepper to taste. Mix well.

4. Spoon the quinoa mixture evenly into the hollowed-out bell peppers.

5. If desired, top the stuffed peppers with shredded cheese.

6. Bake the stuffed peppers for 25-30 minutes, or until the peppers are tender and the filling is heated through.

7. Remove the stuffed peppers from the oven and let them cool for a few minutes before serving.

Serve the Quinoa Stuffed Bell Peppers warm, garnished with additional parsley or feta cheese if desired.

*Enjoy this delicious and nutritious vegetarian dish! The combination of the quinoa, black beans, and fresh vegetables makes for a flavorful and satisfying stuffed pepper.*

# 59. Tofu and vegetable pho

**Ingredients:**
- 8 cups vegetable broth
- 3 whole star anise
- 3 whole cloves
- 1 cinnamon stick
- 1 tablespoon grated fresh ginger
- 1 tablespoon soy sauce
- 1 teaspoon brown sugar
- 8 oz firm or extra-firm tofu, cubed
- 8 oz rice noodles
- 2 cups thinly sliced mixed vegetables (such as carrots, cabbage, bean sprouts, mushrooms)
- 1/4 cup chopped fresh cilantro
- 2 green onions, thinly sliced
- Lime wedges for serving

**Instructions**:

1. In a large pot, combine the vegetable broth, star anise, cloves, cinnamon stick, grated ginger, soy sauce, and brown sugar. Bring to a boil over high heat.

2. Reduce the heat to medium-low and let the broth simmer for 15-20 minutes to allow the flavors to infuse.

3. Add the cubed tofu and rice noodles to the simmering broth. Cook for 5-7 minutes, until the noodles are tender.

4. Stir in the sliced vegetables and cook for 2-3 minutes more, until the vegetables are crisp-tender.

5. Remove the star anise, cloves, and cinnamon stick from the broth.

6. Ladle the pho into bowls and top with the chopped cilantro and sliced green onions.

7. Serve the Tofu and Vegetable Pho immediately, with lime wedges on the side.

***Enjoy this delicious and nourishing vegetarian pho! The combination of the flavorful broth, tender tofu, and fresh vegetables makes for a comforting and satisfying meal.***

# 60. Stuffed acorn squash with wild rice and cranberries

**Ingredients:**
- 2 acorn squash, halved and seeded
- 1 cup cooked wild rice
- 1/2 cup dried cranberries
- 1/4 cup chopped pecans
- 2 tablespoons maple syrup
- 1 teaspoon ground cinnamon
- 1/4 teaspoon ground nutmeg
- Salt and pepper to taste
- 2 tablespoons olive oil

**Instructions:**

1. Preheat your oven to 400°F (200°C).

2. Place the acorn squash halves cut-side up on a baking sheet. Brush the insides with olive oil and season with salt and pepper.

3. Bake the squash for 30-40 minutes, or until tender when pierced with a fork.

4. In a medium bowl, combine the cooked wild rice, dried cranberries, chopped pecans, maple syrup, cinnamon, and nutmeg. Season with salt and pepper to taste.

5. Scoop the wild rice mixture into the baked acorn squash halves, dividing it evenly.

6. Return the stuffed squash to the oven and bake for an additional 15-20 minutes, or until the filling is heated through and the squash is very tender.

7. Serve the Stuffed Acorn Squash with Wild Rice and Cranberries warm, garnished with extra pecans or cranberries if desired.

*Enjoy this delicious and festive stuffed acorn squash dish! The combination of the sweet and nutty wild rice, tart cranberries, and warm spices is simply delightful.*

# 61. Vegetable and tofu stir-fry with peanut sauce

**Ingredients**:
- 1 block (14 oz) firm or extra-firm tofu, cubed
- 2 tablespoons vegetable oil
- 3 cloves garlic, minced
- 1 inch fresh ginger, grated
- 1 red bell pepper, sliced
- 1 cup broccoli florets
- 1 cup sliced mushrooms
- 1 cup snow peas or snap peas
- 2 green onions, sliced
- 1/4 cup creamy peanut butter
- 2 tablespoons soy sauce
- 1 tablespoon rice vinegar
- 1 tablespoon honey or maple syrup
- 1 teaspoon sesame oil
- 1/4 cup water or vegetable broth
- Salt and pepper to taste
- Chopped peanuts and cilantro for garnish (optional)

**Instructions**:

1. In a large skillet or wok, heat the vegetable oil over medium-high heat. Add the cubed tofu and cook, stirring occasionally, until lightly browned on all sides, about 5-7 minutes. Transfer the tofu to a plate.

2. In the same skillet, add the minced garlic and grated ginger. Cook for 1 minute, stirring constantly, until fragrant.

3. Add the sliced bell pepper, broccoli, mushrooms, and snow peas to the skillet. Stir-fry for 3-5 minutes, until the vegetables are crisp-tender.

4. In a small bowl, whisk together the peanut butter, soy sauce, rice vinegar, honey, sesame oil, and water or broth until well combined.

5. Add the cooked tofu and the peanut sauce to the skillet with the vegetables. Toss everything together and cook for 2-3 minutes, until the sauce has thickened and the tofu is heated through.

6. Remove from heat and stir in the sliced green onions. Season with salt and pepper to taste.

7. Serve the Vegetable and Tofu Stir-Fry with Peanut Sauce over rice or noodles. Garnish with chopped peanuts and fresh cilantro, if desired.

***Enjoy this flavorful and nutritious vegetable and tofu stir-fry with the creamy peanut sauce!***

# 62. Stuffed portobello mushrooms with spinach and quinoa

**Ingredients:**
- 4 large portobello mushroom caps, stems removed and chopped
- 1 cup cooked quinoa
- 1 cup fresh spinach, chopped
- 1/2 cup crumbled feta cheese
- 2 cloves garlic, minced
- 2 tablespoons olive oil
- 1 teaspoon dried oregano
- Salt and pepper to taste

**Instructions**:
1. Preheat your oven to 400°F (200°C).

2. Gently clean the portobello mushroom caps with a damp cloth. Remove the stems and chop them.

3. In a skillet, heat the olive oil over medium heat. Add the chopped mushroom stems, minced garlic, and sauté for 2-3 minutes until fragrant.

4. Add the chopped spinach to the skillet and cook for 1-2 minutes, until the spinach is wilted.

5. Transfer the spinach and mushroom mixture to a bowl. Add the cooked quinoa and crumbled feta cheese. Season with dried oregano, salt, and pepper. Mix well.

6. Arrange the portobello mushroom caps, gill-side up, on a baking sheet. Spoon the quinoa and spinach mixture evenly into the mushroom caps.

7. Bake the stuffed portobello mushrooms for 15-20 minutes, or until the mushrooms are tender and the filling is heated through.

8. Remove the stuffed mushrooms from the oven and let them cool for a few minutes before serving.

Serve the Stuffed Portobello Mushrooms with Spinach and Quinoa warm, garnished with extra feta cheese or fresh herbs if desired.

*Enjoy this delicious and healthy vegetarian dish! The combination of the earthy mushrooms, nutrient-rich quinoa, and fresh spinach makes for a satisfying and flavorful meal.*

# 63. Quinoa and vegetable bibimbap bowl

**Ingredients**:
- 1 cup uncooked quinoa, rinsed
- 2 cups vegetable broth
- 1 cup shredded carrots
- 1 cup thinly sliced zucchini
- 1 cup thinly sliced mushrooms
- 1 cup baby spinach leaves
- 2 eggs, fried or soft-boiled
- 2 tablespoons sesame seeds
- 2 tablespoons gochujang (Korean chili paste)
- 1 tablespoon sesame oil
- 1 tablespoon rice vinegar
- 1 teaspoon honey
- Salt and pepper to taste

**Instructions:**

1. Cook the quinoa: In a medium saucepan, combine the rinsed quinoa and vegetable broth. Bring to a boil, then reduce heat to low, cover, and simmer for 15-20 minutes, until the quinoa is tender and the liquid is absorbed. Fluff with a fork.

2. Prepare the vegetables: In a large skillet or wok, sauté the carrots, zucchini, and mushrooms over medium-high heat until tender-crisp, about 5-7 minutes. Add the spinach and cook for 1-2 minutes more, until wilted.

3. Make the bibimbap sauce: In a small bowl, whisk together the gochujang, sesame oil, rice vinegar, and honey. Season with salt and pepper to taste.

4. Assemble the bowls: Divide the cooked quinoa among 4 serving bowls. Top each bowl with the sautéed vegetables, a fried or soft-boiled egg, and a drizzle of the bibimbap sauce. Sprinkle with sesame seeds.

5. Serve immediately, allowing each person to mix the ingredients together in their bowl before eating.

*Enjoy this colorful and flavorful Quinoa and Vegetable Bibimbap Bowl! The combination of the nutty quinoa, fresh vegetables, and spicy-sweet bibimbap sauce makes for a delicious and nutritious meal.*

# 64. Chickpea and vegetable curry

**Ingredients:**
- 1 tablespoon olive oil
- 1 onion, diced
- 3 cloves garlic, minced
- 1 tablespoon grated fresh ginger
- 2 teaspoons garam masala
- 1 teaspoon ground cumin
- 1 teaspoon ground coriander
- 1/2 teaspoon ground turmeric
- 1/4 teaspoon cayenne pepper (or to taste)
- 1 (15 oz) can chickpeas, drained and rinsed
- 1 (14 oz) can diced tomatoes
- 1 cup vegetable broth
- 1 medium potato, peeled and diced
- 1 cup cauliflower florets
- 1 cup frozen peas
- 1 cup spinach leaves
- 1/4 cup chopped fresh cilantro
- Salt and pepper to taste
- Cooked basmati rice, for serving

**Instructions:**

1. In a large skillet or Dutch oven, heat the olive oil over medium heat. Add the diced onion and sauté for 5-7 minutes, until translucent.

2. Add the minced garlic and grated ginger to the skillet. Cook for 1 minute, until fragrant.

3. Stir in the garam masala, cumin, coriander, turmeric, and cayenne pepper. Cook for 2-3 minutes, stirring constantly, to toast the spices.

4. Add the drained and rinsed chickpeas, diced tomatoes, and vegetable broth. Bring the mixture to a simmer.

5. Add the diced potato, cauliflower florets, and frozen peas. Simmer for 15-20 minutes, until the vegetables are tender.

6. Stir in the spinach leaves and chopped cilantro. Cook for 2-3 minutes more, until the spinach is wilted.

7. Season the curry with salt and pepper to taste. Serve the Chickpea and Vegetable Curry over cooked basmati rice. Garnish with additional cilantro if desired.

***Enjoy this flavorful and nourishing chickpea and vegetable curry! The combination of spices, vegetables, and protein-rich chickpeas makes for a satisfying and comforting meal.***

# 65. Lentil and vegetable pot pie

**Ingredients**:
*For the Filling:*
- 1 cup brown or green lentils, rinsed
- 4 cups vegetable broth
- 1 tablespoon olive oil
- 1 onion, diced
- 3 carrots, peeled and diced
- 2 celery stalks, diced
- 3 cloves garlic, minced
- 1 teaspoon dried thyme
- 1 teaspoon dried rosemary
- Salt and pepper to taste

*For the Crust:*
- 1 1/2 cups all-purpose flour
- 1/2 teaspoon salt
- 1/2 cup cold unsalted butter, cubed
- 1/4 cup ice water

**Instructions**:

*1. Make the Filling:*
   - In a medium saucepan, combine the lentils and vegetable broth. Bring to a boil, then reduce heat and simmer for 20-25 minutes, until the lentils are tender. Drain any excess liquid and set aside.
   - In a large skillet, heat the olive oil over medium heat. Add the diced onion, carrots, and celery. Sauté for 5-7 minutes, until the vegetables are softened.
   - Add the minced garlic, dried thyme, and dried rosemary. Cook for 1 minute, until fragrant.
   - Stir in the cooked lentils and season with salt and pepper to taste. Set the filling aside.

*2. Make the Crust:*
   - In a food processor, combine the flour and salt. Add the cold cubed butter and pulse until the mixture resembles coarse crumbs.
   - Add the ice water 1 tablespoon at a time, pulsing until the dough just begins to come together.
   - Turn the dough out onto a lightly floured surface and gently shape it into a disk. Wrap in plastic wrap and refrigerate for at least 30 minutes.

*3. Assemble and Bake the Pot Pie:*
   - Preheat your oven to 400°F (200°C).
   - Transfer the lentil and vegetable filling to a 9-inch pie dish or baking dish.
   - Roll out the chilled dough to a size that will fit over the top of the pie dish. Place the dough over the filling, pressing the edges to seal.
   - Cut a few slits in the top of the dough to allow steam to escape.
   - Bake the pot pie for 30-35 minutes, until the crust is golden brown and the filling is bubbling.
   - Let the pot pie cool for 10-15 minutes before serving.

# 66. Stuffed tomatoes with quinoa and spinach

**Ingredients:**
- 6 medium tomatoes
- 1 cup cooked quinoa
- 1 cup fresh spinach, chopped
- 1/2 cup crumbled feta cheese
- 2 tablespoons chopped fresh basil
- 2 cloves garlic, minced
- 1 tablespoon olive oil
- Salt and pepper to taste

**Instructions**:

1. Preheat your oven to 375°F (190°C).

2. Cut the tops off the tomatoes and scoop out the insides, reserving the pulp. Chop the tomato pulp.

3. In a medium bowl, combine the chopped tomato pulp, cooked quinoa, chopped spinach, crumbled feta cheese, chopped basil, and minced garlic. Mix well and season with salt and pepper to taste.

4. Stuff the tomato shells with the quinoa and spinach mixture, packing it in tightly.

5. Place the stuffed tomatoes in a baking dish. Drizzle the tops with the olive oil.

6. Bake the stuffed tomatoes for 20-25 minutes, or until the tomatoes are softened and the filling is heated through.

7. Serve the stuffed tomatoes warm, garnished with additional fresh basil if desired.

***Enjoy these delicious and nutritious Stuffed Tomatoes with Quinoa and Spinach! The combination of the juicy tomatoes, fluffy quinoa, and fresh spinach and herbs makes for a flavorful and satisfying vegetarian dish.***

# 67. Tofu and vegetable pad Thai

**Ingredients:**
- 8 oz rice noodles
- 2 tablespoons vegetable oil
- 1 block (14 oz) firm or extra-firm tofu, cubed
- 2 cloves garlic, minced
- 1 cup thinly sliced carrots
- 1 cup bean sprouts
- 1 cup chopped green cabbage
- 2 green onions, sliced
- 1/4 cup chopped roasted peanuts
- 2 tablespoons chopped fresh cilantro

*For the Sauce:*
- 3 tablespoons fish sauce (or soy sauce for a vegetarian/vegan version)
- 2 tablespoons lime juice
- 2 tablespoons brown sugar
- 1 tablespoon soy sauce
- 1 teaspoon Sriracha or other hot sauce (optional)

**Instructions:**
1. Soak the rice noodles in hot water for 15-20 minutes, until softened. Drain and set aside.

2. In a small bowl, whisk together all the sauce ingredients and set aside.

3. In a large skillet or wok, heat the vegetable oil over medium-high heat. Add the cubed tofu and cook, stirring occasionally, until lightly browned on all sides, about 5-7 minutes. Transfer the tofu to a plate.

4. In the same skillet, add the minced garlic and sauté for 1 minute until fragrant.

5. Add the sliced carrots, bean sprouts, and chopped cabbage to the skillet. Stir-fry for 3-5 minutes, until the vegetables are crisp-tender.

6. Add the cooked rice noodles and the prepared sauce to the skillet. Toss everything together until the noodles are well coated and heated through, about 2-3 minutes.

7. Stir in the cooked tofu and the sliced green onions. Cook for 1-2 minutes more.

8. Remove from heat and garnish the pad Thai with chopped roasted peanuts and fresh cilantro.

# 68. Stuffed mushrooms with quinoa and spinach

**Ingredients**:
- 12 large mushrooms, stems removed and chopped
- 1 cup cooked quinoa
- 1 cup fresh spinach, chopped
- 1/4 cup grated Parmesan cheese
- 2 cloves garlic, minced
- 2 tablespoons olive oil
- 1 teaspoon dried thyme
- Salt and pepper to taste

**Instructions:**

1. Preheat your oven to 375°F (190°C).

2. Clean the mushroom caps with a damp cloth and remove the stems. Finely chop the stems.

3. In a skillet, heat the olive oil over medium heat. Add the chopped mushroom stems and minced garlic. Sauté for 2-3 minutes until fragrant.

4. Add the chopped spinach to the skillet and cook for 1-2 minutes, until the spinach is wilted. Remove from heat and let cool slightly.

5. In a medium bowl, combine the sautéed mushroom stem and spinach mixture with the cooked quinoa and grated Parmesan cheese. Season with dried thyme, salt, and pepper.

6. Arrange the mushroom caps, gill-side up, on a baking sheet. Spoon the quinoa and spinach filling into the mushroom caps, dividing it evenly.

7. Bake the stuffed mushrooms for 15-20 minutes, or until the mushrooms are tender and the filling is heated through.

8. Remove the stuffed mushrooms from the oven and let them cool for a few minutes before serving.

Serve the Stuffed Mushrooms with Quinoa and Spinach warm, garnished with additional Parmesan cheese or fresh herbs if desired.

*Enjoy this delightful vegetarian appetizer or side dish! The combination of the earthy mushrooms, nutty quinoa, and fresh spinach makes for a flavorful and satisfying stuffed mushroom.*

# 69. Tofu and vegetable sushi bowl

**Ingredients:**
- 1 cup uncooked short-grain brown rice
- 2 cups water
- 1/4 cup rice vinegar
- 2 tablespoons sugar
- 1 teaspoon salt
- 1 block (14 oz) firm or extra-firm tofu, cubed
- 1 tablespoon sesame oil
- 1 carrot, julienned or shredded
- 1 cucumber, julienned or shredded
- 1 avocado, sliced
- 1 cup shredded purple cabbage
- 2 tablespoons toasted sesame seeds
- 2 tablespoons chopped fresh cilantro
- Soy sauce, for serving

**Instructions:**

1. Cook the brown rice: In a medium saucepan, combine the brown rice and water. Bring to a boil, then reduce heat to low, cover, and simmer for 25-30 minutes, until the rice is tender and the water is absorbed. Fluff with a fork.

2. Make the sushi rice: In a small bowl, whisk together the rice vinegar, sugar, and salt until the sugar has dissolved. Pour the vinegar mixture over the cooked brown rice and gently mix to combine. Set aside.

3. Cook the tofu: In a large skillet, heat the sesame oil over medium-high heat. Add the cubed tofu and cook, stirring occasionally, until lightly browned on all sides, about 5-7 minutes.

4. Assemble the sushi bowls: Divide the sushi rice among 4 serving bowls. Top each bowl with the cooked tofu, julienned carrots, julienned cucumber, sliced avocado, and shredded purple cabbage.

5. Sprinkle the sushi bowls with toasted sesame seeds and chopped fresh cilantro. Serve the Tofu and Vegetable Sushi Bowls with soy sauce on the side for drizzling or dipping.

***Enjoy this colorful and flavorful Tofu and Vegetable Sushi Bowl! The combination of the seasoned sushi rice, crisp vegetables, and savory tofu makes for a delicious and satisfying meal. Feel free to adjust the toppings to your liking.***

# 70. Vegan bibimbap bowl

**Ingredients:**
- 1 cup cooked brown rice
- 1 cup shredded carrots
- 1 cup shredded zucchini
- 1 cup shredded purple cabbage
- 1 cup baby spinach leaves
- 1 cup cooked edamame
- 1 avocado, sliced
- 2 tablespoons toasted sesame seeds
- 2 tablespoons gochujang (Korean chili paste)
- 1 tablespoon sesame oil
- 1 tablespoon rice vinegar
- 1 teaspoon maple syrup
- Salt and pepper to taste

**Instructions:**

1. Prepare the rice according to package instructions and set aside.

2. In a large bowl, arrange the cooked brown rice, shredded carrots, shredded zucchini, shredded purple cabbage, baby spinach leaves, and cooked edamame.

3. Top the bowl with sliced avocado.

4. In a small bowl, whisk together the gochujang, sesame oil, rice vinegar, and maple syrup. Season with salt and pepper to taste.

5. Drizzle the gochujang sauce over the bibimbap bowl.

6. Sprinkle the toasted sesame seeds over the top.

7. Serve the Vegan Bibimbap Bowl immediately, allowing each person to mix the ingredients together in their bowl before eating.

Enjoy this colorful, flavorful, and nutritious Vegan Bibimbap Bowl! The combination of the nutty brown rice, fresh vegetables, and the spicy-sweet gochujang sauce makes for a delicious and satisfying plant-based meal.

*Feel free to adjust the vegetable toppings to your liking. You can also add other toppings like sautéed mushrooms, crispy tofu, or a fried egg (if not vegan) for extra protein and flavor.*

# 71. Lentil and vegetable biryani

**Ingredients:**
- 1 cup brown or green lentils, rinsed
- 2 cups vegetable broth
- 2 tablespoons olive oil
- 1 onion, diced
- 3 cloves garlic, minced
- 1 tablespoon grated fresh ginger
- 2 teaspoons garam masala
- 1 teaspoon ground cumin
- 1 teaspoon ground coriander
- 1/2 teaspoon ground turmeric
- 1/4 teaspoon cayenne pepper (or to taste)
- 1 cup diced potatoes
- 1 cup cauliflower florets
- 1 cup frozen peas
- 1 cup diced tomatoes
- 1/4 cup chopped fresh cilantro
- 1 cup basmati rice, cooked according to package instructions
- Salt and pepper to taste

**Instructions:**

1. In a medium saucepan, combine the lentils and vegetable broth. Bring to a boil, then reduce heat and simmer for 20-25 minutes, until the lentils are tender. Drain any excess liquid and set aside.

2. In a large skillet or Dutch oven, heat the olive oil over medium heat. Add the diced onion and sauté for 5-7 minutes, until translucent.

3. Add the minced garlic and grated ginger to the skillet. Cook for 1 minute, until fragrant.

4. Stir in the garam masala, cumin, coriander, turmeric, and cayenne pepper. Cook for 2-3 minutes, stirring constantly, to toast the spices.

5. Add the diced potatoes, cauliflower florets, frozen peas, and diced tomatoes to the skillet. Sauté for 5-7 minutes, until the vegetables are tender.

6. Stir in the cooked lentils and chopped fresh cilantro. Season with salt and pepper to taste.

7. Serve the Lentil and Vegetable Biryani over the cooked basmati rice.

Garnish the biryani with additional chopped cilantro, if desired.

**Enjoy this flavorful and nourishing Lentil and Vegetable Biryani! The combination of spices, vegetables, and protein-rich lentils makes for a satisfying and comforting vegetarian dish. Let me know if you have any other questions.**

# 72. Vegetable curry with tempeh

**Ingredients:**
- 1 block (8 oz) tempeh, cut into cubes
- 2 tablespoons coconut oil
- 1 onion, diced
- 3 cloves garlic, minced
- 1 tablespoon grated fresh ginger
- 2 teaspoons curry powder
- 1 teaspoon ground cumin
- 1 teaspoon ground coriander
- 1/2 teaspoon ground turmeric
- 1/4 teaspoon cayenne pepper (or to taste)
- 1 cup diced potatoes
- 1 cup cauliflower florets
- 1 cup diced carrots
- 1 cup diced bell pepper
- 1 (14 oz) can diced tomatoes
- 1 (13.5 oz) can coconut milk
- 1 cup frozen peas
- 1/4 cup chopped fresh cilantro
- Salt and pepper to taste
- Cooked basmati rice, for serving

**Instructions:**

1. In a large skillet or wok, heat the coconut oil over medium-high heat. Add the cubed tempeh and cook, stirring occasionally, until lightly browned on all sides, about 5-7 minutes. Transfer the tempeh to a plate.

2. In the same skillet, add the diced onion and sauté for 5-7 minutes, until translucent.

3. Add the minced garlic and grated ginger to the skillet. Cook for 1 minute, until fragrant.

4. Stir in the curry powder, cumin, coriander, turmeric, and cayenne pepper. Cook for 2-3 minutes, stirring constantly, to toast the spices.

5. Add the diced potatoes, cauliflower florets, diced carrots, and diced bell pepper to the skillet. Sauté for 5-7 minutes, until the vegetables are starting to soften.

6. Pour in the diced tomatoes and coconut milk. Bring the mixture to a simmer and cook for 15-20 minutes, until the vegetables are tender.

7. Stir in the cooked tempeh and frozen peas. Cook for 5 minutes more, until the peas are heated through.

8. Remove from heat and stir in the chopped fresh cilantro. Season with salt and pepper to taste. Serve the Vegetable Curry with Tempeh over cooked basmati rice.

***Enjoy this flavorful and nourishing vegetable curry! The combination of the aromatic spices, creamy coconut milk, and protein-rich tempeh makes for a satisfying and comforting meal.***

# 73. Stuffed bell peppers with lentils and quinoa

**Ingredients:**
- 6 bell peppers (any color)
- 1 cup cooked lentils
- 1 cup cooked quinoa
- 1 small onion, diced
- 2 cloves garlic, minced
- 1 cup diced tomatoes
- 1 tsp cumin
- 1 tsp oregano
- Salt and pepper to taste
- Shredded cheese (optional)

**Instructions**:

1. Preheat oven to 375°F.

2. Cut the tops off the bell peppers and remove the seeds and membranes. Place the peppers in a baking dish.

3. In a bowl, mix together the cooked lentils, quinoa, onion, garlic, tomatoes, cumin, oregano, salt and pepper.

4. Stuff the mixture into the hollowed out bell peppers.

5. If desired, top the stuffed peppers with shredded cheese.

6. Bake for 30-35 minutes, until the peppers are tender.

7. Serve hot.

The lentils and quinoa provide a hearty, protein-packed filling for the bell peppers. You can adjust the seasonings to your taste. Enjoy!

# 74. Tofu and vegetable stir-fry with cashews

**Ingredients**:
- 1 block (14 oz) extra-firm tofu, cubed
- 2 tbsp vegetable oil
- 1 red bell pepper, sliced
- 1 cup broccoli florets
- 1 cup sliced mushrooms
- 1 cup snow peas or snap peas
- 3 cloves garlic, minced
- 1 tbsp grated ginger
- 2 tbsp soy sauce
- 1 tbsp rice vinegar
- 1 tsp sesame oil
- 1/4 cup roasted cashews

**Instructions**:
1. Press the tofu for 15-30 minutes to remove excess moisture. Cut into 1-inch cubes.

2. Heat the vegetable oil in a large skillet or wok over high heat. Add the tofu and cook for 2-3 minutes per side until lightly browned. Remove tofu from pan and set aside.

3. Add the bell pepper, broccoli, mushrooms and snow peas to the pan. Stir-fry for 3-4 minutes until vegetables are tender-crisp.

4. Add the garlic and ginger and cook for 1 minute until fragrant.

5. Return the tofu to the pan. Add the soy sauce, rice vinegar and sesame oil. Toss everything together and cook for 2-3 more minutes.

6. Remove from heat and stir in the roasted cashews.

7. Serve immediately over rice or noodles.

*The combination of crispy tofu, fresh vegetables and crunchy cashews makes this a delicious and nutritious stir-fry. Adjust the sauce ingredients to your taste.*

# 75. Chickpea and vegetable tagine

**Ingredients:**
- 2 tbsp olive oil
- 1 onion, diced
- 3 cloves garlic, minced
- 1 tsp ground cumin
- 1 tsp ground coriander
- 1 tsp paprika
- 1/2 tsp ground cinnamon
- 1/4 tsp cayenne pepper (optional)
- 1 (15oz) can chickpeas, drained and rinsed
- 1 (14oz) can diced tomatoes
- 1 cup vegetable broth
- 1 medium sweet potato, peeled and cubed
- 1 cup cauliflower florets
- 1 cup green beans, trimmed and cut into 1-inch pieces
- Salt and pepper to taste
- Chopped cilantro for garnish

**Instructions:**

1. In a large pot or Dutch oven, heat the olive oil over medium heat. Add the onion and sauté for 5 minutes until translucent.

2. Add the garlic, cumin, coriander, paprika, cinnamon and cayenne (if using). Cook for 1 minute until fragrant.

3. Stir in the chickpeas, diced tomatoes, vegetable broth, sweet potato, cauliflower and green beans. Season with salt and pepper.

4. Bring the mixture to a simmer, then reduce heat to medium-low. Cover and cook for 20-25 minutes, until the vegetables are tender.

5. Taste and adjust seasonings as needed.

6. Serve the tagine warm, garnished with chopped cilantro. Can be served over couscous or rice.

**The blend of spices creates a delicious Moroccan-inspired flavor in this hearty vegetable and chickpea stew. Feel free to substitute other vegetables as desired.**

# 76. Stuffed sweet potatoes with quinoa and black beans

**Ingredients:**
- 4 medium sweet potatoes
- 1 cup cooked quinoa
- 1 (15oz) can black beans, drained and rinsed
- 1 cup corn kernels (fresh or frozen)
- 1 red bell pepper, diced
- 1 jalapeño, seeded and minced (optional)
- 2 cloves garlic, minced
- 1 tsp ground cumin
- 1 tsp chili powder
- Salt and pepper to taste
- Chopped cilantro for garnish
- Shredded cheese (optional)

**Instructions:**

1. Preheat oven to 400°F. Pierce the sweet potatoes several times with a fork. Bake for 45-60 minutes, until very soft when squeezed.

2. Let the sweet potatoes cool slightly, then slice them in half lengthwise. Scoop out the flesh into a bowl, leaving a thin layer attached to the skin.

3. In the bowl with the sweet potato flesh, mix together the cooked quinoa, black beans, corn, bell pepper, jalapeño (if using), garlic, cumin, chili powder, salt and pepper.

4. Stuff the sweet potato skins with the quinoa and black bean mixture.

5. Place the stuffed sweet potatoes on a baking sheet. Bake for 10-15 minutes, until heated through.

6. Remove from oven and top with chopped cilantro and shredded cheese, if desired.

7. Serve warm.

*The combination of sweet potatoes, quinoa, black beans and veggies makes these stuffed sweet potatoes a nutritious and flavorful meal. Adjust the spices to your taste.*

# 77. Vegan sushi rolls with tofu and avocado

**Ingredients:**
- 1 cup sushi rice
- 2 tbsp rice vinegar
- 1 tsp sugar
- 1/2 tsp salt
- 1 block extra-firm tofu, pressed and cut into thin strips
- 1 avocado, sliced
- 1 carrot, julienned
- 1 cucumber, julienned
- Nori seaweed sheets
- Soy sauce, for serving

**Instructions:**

1. Cook the sushi rice according to package instructions. Transfer to a large bowl and stir in the rice vinegar, sugar and salt. Let cool.

2. Place a nori sheet shiny-side down on a bamboo sushi mat. Spread about 3/4 cup of the seasoned sushi rice evenly over the nori, leaving a 1-inch border at the top.

3. Arrange a few strips of tofu, avocado, carrot and cucumber in a line across the center of the rice.

4. Starting from the bottom, use the sushi mat to tightly roll up the nori sheet around the fillings. Moisten the top edge with water to seal the roll.

5. Repeat with remaining nori sheets and fillings to make 4-6 rolls total.

6. Using a very sharp knife, slice each roll into 6-8 pieces.

7. Serve the vegan sushi rolls immediately with soy sauce for dipping.

Tips:
- Use a bamboo sushi mat to help roll the sushi tightly.
- Wet your hands when handling the sticky sushi rice.
- Experiment with different veggie fillings like spinach, bell peppers or pickled ginger.

***Enjoy these fresh and flavorful vegan sushi rolls!***

# 78. Lentil and vegetable curry

**Ingredients:**
- 1 cup dried brown or green lentils, rinsed
- 1 tbsp olive oil
- 1 onion, diced
- 3 cloves garlic, minced
- 1 tbsp grated fresh ginger
- 2 tsp garam masala
- 1 tsp ground cumin
- 1 tsp ground coriander
- 1/2 tsp turmeric
- 1/4 tsp cayenne pepper (optional)
- 1 (14oz) can diced tomatoes
- 1 cup vegetable broth
- 1 medium potato, peeled and cubed
- 1 cup cauliflower florets
- 1 cup frozen peas
- Salt and pepper to taste
- Chopped cilantro for garnish

**Instructions:**

1. In a large pot, cover the lentils with water and bring to a boil. Reduce heat and simmer for 15-20 minutes until tender. Drain and set aside.

2. In the same pot, heat the olive oil over medium heat. Add the onion and sauté for 5 minutes until translucent.

3. Stir in the garlic, ginger, garam masala, cumin, coriander, turmeric and cayenne (if using). Cook for 1 minute until fragrant.

4. Add the diced tomatoes, vegetable broth, potato, cauliflower and peas. Bring to a simmer.

5. Stir in the cooked lentils and season with salt and pepper to taste.

6. Reduce heat to medium-low and let the curry simmer for 15-20 minutes, until the vegetables are tender.

7. Serve the lentil and vegetable curry warm, garnished with chopped cilantro. Can be served over rice or with naan bread.

***The blend of aromatic spices creates a delicious Indian-inspired curry. Feel free to adjust the spices to your preference.***

# 79. Stuffed bell peppers with quinoa and chickpeas

**Ingredients:**
- 6 bell peppers (any color)
- 1 cup cooked quinoa
- 1 (15oz) can chickpeas, drained and rinsed
- 1 small onion, diced
- 2 cloves garlic, minced
- 1 cup diced tomatoes
- 1 tsp ground cumin
- 1 tsp dried oregano
- 1/4 tsp red pepper flakes (optional)
- Salt and pepper to taste
- Shredded cheese (optional)

**Instructions:**
1. Preheat oven to 375°F.

2. Cut the tops off the bell peppers and remove the seeds and membranes. Place the peppers in a baking dish.

3. In a bowl, combine the cooked quinoa, chickpeas, onion, garlic, diced tomatoes, cumin, oregano, red pepper flakes (if using), salt and pepper.

4. Stuff the quinoa and chickpea mixture into the hollowed out bell peppers.

5. If desired, top the stuffed peppers with shredded cheese.

6. Bake for 30-35 minutes, until the peppers are tender.

7. Serve hot.

The quinoa and chickpeas provide a hearty, protein-packed filling for the bell peppers. The tomatoes, onion and spices add great flavor. You can adjust the seasonings to your taste.

**These stuffed peppers make a delicious and nutritious vegetarian main dish. Serve them with a side salad or roasted vegetables for a complete meal.**

# 80. Tofu and vegetable bibimbap bowl

**Ingredients:**
- 1 block extra-firm tofu, pressed and cubed
- 2 tbsp sesame oil, divided
- 2 cups cooked brown rice
- 1 cup shredded carrots
- 1 cup shredded spinach
- 1 cup bean sprouts
- 1 cup sliced mushrooms
- 2 scallions, sliced
- 2 tbsp gochujang (Korean chili paste)
- 2 tbsp soy sauce
- 1 tsp sesame seeds
- Salt and pepper to taste
- Fried egg (optional)

**Instructions:**

1. In a large skillet, heat 1 tbsp sesame oil over medium-high heat. Add the tofu cubes and cook for 5-7 minutes, turning occasionally, until lightly browned on all sides. Remove tofu from pan and set aside.

2. In the same pan, heat the remaining 1 tbsp sesame oil. Add the carrots, spinach, bean sprouts and mushrooms. Sauté for 3-4 minutes until vegetables are tender-crisp.

3. In a large bowl, layer the cooked brown rice, sautéed vegetables, and cooked tofu.

4. In a small bowl, whisk together the gochujang, soy sauce and sesame seeds.

5. Drizzle the gochujang sauce over the bibimbap bowl. Top with sliced scallions and a fried egg, if desired.

6. Season with salt and pepper to taste.

7. Serve the bibimbap bowl warm, mixing everything together before eating.

*This colorful and flavorful bibimbap bowl is packed with nutritious vegetables, protein-rich tofu, and a delicious gochujang sauce. Adjust the spice level to your preference.*

# 81. Lentil and vegetable birria tacos

**Ingredients:**
***For the Birria Filling:***
- 1 cup dried brown or green lentils, rinsed
- 1 onion, diced
- 3 cloves garlic, minced
- 2 tsp chili powder
- 1 tsp ground cumin
- 1 tsp dried oregano
- 1 tsp smoked paprika
- 1/4 tsp ground cinnamon
- 1 (14oz) can diced tomatoes
- 1 cup vegetable broth
- Salt and pepper to taste

***For the Tacos:***
- 12-16 corn tortillas
- Shredded cabbage or lettuce
- Diced onion
- Chopped cilantro
- Lime wedges
- Queso fresco or shredded cheese (optional)

**Instructions:**
1. In a large pot, combine the lentils, onion, garlic, chili powder, cumin, oregano, paprika, cinnamon, diced tomatoes and vegetable broth. Bring to a boil.

2. Reduce heat to medium-low and simmer for 20-25 minutes, until the lentils are very soft. Season with salt and pepper.

3. Using a potato masher or the back of a spoon, roughly mash the lentil mixture to create a thick, stew-like consistency.

4. Heat the corn tortillas according to package instructions.

5. To assemble the tacos, place a spoonful of the lentil birria filling into each tortilla. Top with shredded cabbage, diced onion, chopped cilantro and a squeeze of lime juice.

6. Optionally, you can also top the tacos with crumbled queso fresco or shredded cheese. Serve the lentil birria tacos immediately.

# 82. Quinoa stuffed bell peppers

**Ingredients:**
- 6 bell peppers (any color)
- 1 cup cooked quinoa
- 1 (15oz) can black beans, drained and rinsed
- 1 cup diced tomatoes
- 1/2 cup diced onion
- 2 cloves garlic, minced
- 1 tsp ground cumin
- 1 tsp dried oregano
- 1/4 tsp cayenne pepper (optional)
- Salt and pepper to taste
- Shredded cheese (optional)

**Instructions:**

1. Preheat oven to 375°F.

2. Cut the tops off the bell peppers and remove the seeds and membranes. Place the peppers in a baking dish.

3. In a bowl, combine the cooked quinoa, black beans, diced tomatoes, onion, garlic, cumin, oregano, cayenne (if using), salt and pepper.

4. Stuff the quinoa and vegetable mixture into the hollowed out bell peppers.

5. If desired, top the stuffed peppers with shredded cheese.

6. Bake for 30-35 minutes, until the peppers are tender.

7. Serve hot.

The quinoa and black beans provide a hearty, protein-packed filling for the bell peppers. The tomatoes, onion and spices add great flavor. You can adjust the seasonings to your taste.

**These stuffed peppers make a delicious and nutritious vegetarian main dish. Serve them with a side salad or roasted vegetables for a complete meal.**

# 83. Tofu and vegetable pho

**Ingredients:**
- 8 cups vegetable broth
- 3 whole star anise
- 3 whole cloves
- 1 cinnamon stick
- 1 tbsp grated ginger
- 2 tsp soy sauce
- 1 block extra-firm tofu, cubed
- 8 oz rice noodles
- 2 cups sliced mushrooms
- 1 cup bean sprouts
- 1 cup shredded carrots
- 1 cup chopped spinach or bok choy
- 2 green onions, sliced
- Lime wedges, for serving
- Chopped cilantro, for serving

**Instructions:**

1. In a large pot, combine the vegetable broth, star anise, cloves, cinnamon stick and grated ginger. Bring to a boil, then reduce heat and simmer for 15 minutes.

2. Stir in the soy sauce and tofu. Simmer for 5 more minutes.

3. Meanwhile, prepare the rice noodles according to package instructions. Drain and set aside.

4. Add the mushrooms, bean sprouts, carrots and spinach/bok choy to the broth. Simmer for 2-3 minutes until vegetables are tender.

5. To serve, place the cooked rice noodles in the bottom of a bowl. Ladle the hot broth and vegetables over the noodles.

6. Top each bowl with sliced green onions, a squeeze of lime juice, and chopped cilantro.

**The aromatic broth, chewy rice noodles, crisp vegetables and tender tofu make this a nourishing and flavorful vegetarian pho. Adjust the vegetables as desired.**

# 84. Stuffed acorn squash with quinoa and cranberries

**Ingredients:**
- 2 acorn squash, halved and seeded
- 1 cup cooked quinoa
- 1/2 cup dried cranberries
- 1/4 cup chopped pecans
- 2 tbsp maple syrup
- 1 tsp ground cinnamon
- 1/4 tsp ground nutmeg
- Salt and pepper to taste
- Chopped parsley for garnish (optional)

**Instructions**:

1. Preheat oven to 400°F. Place the acorn squash halves cut-side up on a baking sheet. Bake for 30-40 minutes, until tender when pierced with a fork.

2. In a medium bowl, combine the cooked quinoa, dried cranberries, chopped pecans, maple syrup, cinnamon, nutmeg, salt and pepper.

3. Scoop the quinoa mixture evenly into the baked acorn squash halves.

4. Return the stuffed squash to the oven and bake for an additional 15-20 minutes, until the filling is hot and the squash is very tender.

5. Carefully transfer the stuffed squash halves to a serving plate.

6. Garnish with chopped parsley, if desired.

7. Serve the stuffed acorn squash warm.

The sweet and nutty quinoa filling pairs beautifully with the roasted acorn squash. The dried cranberries add a nice pop of tartness. This makes a lovely vegetarian main dish or side.

**You can adjust the spices and add-ins to your taste. Enjoy this cozy and flavorful stuffed squash!**

# 85. Vegetable and tofu stir-fry with almond sauce

**Ingredients:**
*For the Almond Sauce:*
- 1/2 cup almond butter
- 1/4 cup soy sauce
- 2 tbsp rice vinegar
- 1 tbsp maple syrup
- 1 tsp sesame oil
- 1 clove garlic, minced
- 1/4 tsp red pepper flakes (optional)
- 2-3 tbsp water to thin the sauce

*For the Stir-Fry:*
- 1 block extra-firm tofu, pressed and cubed
- 2 tbsp vegetable oil
- 1 red bell pepper, sliced
- 1 cup broccoli florets
- 1 cup snow peas or snap peas
- 2 cups sliced mushrooms
- 3 cloves garlic, minced
- 1 tbsp grated ginger
- 2 tbsp toasted sliced almonds

**Instructions:**

1. Make the almond sauce: In a small bowl, whisk together the almond butter, soy sauce, rice vinegar, maple syrup, sesame oil, garlic and red pepper flakes (if using). Add water 1 tbsp at a time to thin the sauce to a pourable consistency. Set aside.

2. In a large skillet or wok, heat the vegetable oil over high heat. Add the tofu cubes and cook for 2-3 minutes per side until lightly browned. Remove tofu from pan and set aside.

3. Add the bell pepper, broccoli, snow peas and mushrooms to the pan. Stir-fry for 3-4 minutes until vegetables are tender-crisp.

4. Stir in the garlic and ginger and cook for 1 minute until fragrant.

5. Return the tofu to the pan and pour in the almond sauce. Toss everything together to coat evenly.

6. Serve the vegetable and tofu stir-fry immediately, garnished with the toasted sliced almonds.

The creamy almond sauce adds a delicious nutty flavor to this veggie-packed stir-fry. Adjust the amount of red pepper flakes to control the heat level.

*Serve this dish over rice or noodles for a complete meal.*

# 86. Stuffed portobello mushrooms with spinach and rice

**Ingredients:**
- 4 large portobello mushroom caps, stems removed and chopped
- 1 tbsp olive oil
- 1 small onion, diced
- 2 cloves garlic, minced
- 2 cups baby spinach, chopped
- 1 cup cooked brown rice
- 1/4 cup grated Parmesan cheese
- 1 tsp dried oregano
- Salt and pepper to taste
- Shredded mozzarella cheese for topping (optional)

**Instructions**:
1. Preheat oven to 400°F. Arrange the portobello mushroom caps, gill-side up, on a baking sheet.

2. In a skillet, heat the olive oil over medium heat. Add the chopped mushroom stems, onion and garlic. Sauté for 3-4 minutes until softened.

3. Stir in the chopped spinach and cook for 1-2 minutes until wilted.

4. Remove the skillet from heat and stir in the cooked brown rice, Parmesan cheese, oregano, salt and pepper.

5. Spoon the spinach and rice mixture evenly into the portobello mushroom caps.

6. If desired, top the stuffed mushrooms with shredded mozzarella cheese.

7. Bake for 15-20 minutes, until the mushrooms are tender and the filling is hot.

8. Serve the stuffed portobello mushrooms warm.

The combination of earthy mushrooms, nutrient-rich spinach, and nutty brown rice makes these stuffed portobellos a delicious and satisfying vegetarian main dish. The Parmesan cheese adds a nice savory flavor.

***Feel free to adjust the fillings to your taste. These would also work well as a side dish.***

# 87. Quinoa and vegetable bibimbap bowl

**Ingredients:**
- 1 cup cooked quinoa
- 1 cup shredded carrots
- 1 cup shredded spinach
- 1 cup bean sprouts
- 1 cup sliced mushrooms
- 2 scallions, sliced
- 2 tbsp gochujang (Korean chili paste)
- 2 tbsp soy sauce
- 1 tsp sesame seeds
- Salt and pepper to taste
- Fried egg (optional)

**Instructions:**

1. In a large bowl, layer the cooked quinoa, shredded carrots, spinach, bean sprouts and sliced mushrooms.

2. In a small bowl, whisk together the gochujang, soy sauce and sesame seeds to make the bibimbap sauce.

3. Drizzle the gochujang sauce over the quinoa and vegetable bowl.

4. Top with sliced scallions and a fried egg, if desired.

5. Season the bibimbap bowl with salt and pepper to taste.

6. Serve the quinoa and vegetable bibimbap warm, mixing everything together before eating.

This colorful and flavorful bibimbap bowl is packed with nutritious vegetables, protein-rich quinoa, and a delicious gochujang sauce. The fried egg adds a nice richness.

You can adjust the vegetables based on your preferences. The gochujang sauce provides a tasty Korean-inspired flavor.

***This makes a great vegetarian main dish or side. Enjoy!***

# 88. Chickpea and vegetable curry

**Ingredients:**
- 2 tbsp olive oil
- 1 onion, diced
- 3 cloves garlic, minced
- 1 tbsp grated fresh ginger
- 2 tsp garam masala
- 1 tsp ground cumin
- 1 tsp ground coriander
- 1/2 tsp turmeric
- 1/4 tsp cayenne pepper (optional)
- 1 (15oz) can chickpeas, drained and rinsed
- 1 (14oz) can diced tomatoes
- 1 cup vegetable broth
- 1 medium potato, peeled and cubed
- 1 cup cauliflower florets
- 1 cup frozen peas
- Salt and pepper to taste
- Chopped cilantro for garnish

**Instructions:**
1. In a large pot, heat the olive oil over medium heat. Add the onion and sauté for 5 minutes until translucent.

2. Stir in the garlic, ginger, garam masala, cumin, coriander, turmeric and cayenne (if using). Cook for 1 minute until fragrant.

3. Add the chickpeas, diced tomatoes, vegetable broth, potato, cauliflower and peas. Bring to a simmer.

4. Reduce heat to medium-low and let the curry simmer for 15-20 minutes, until the vegetables are tender.

5. Season with salt and pepper to taste.

6. Serve the chickpea and vegetable curry warm, garnished with chopped cilantro. Can be served over rice or with naan bread.

The blend of aromatic spices creates a delicious Indian-inspired curry. The chickpeas provide protein while the vegetables add fiber and nutrients. Adjust the spices to your preference.

# 89. Lentil and vegetable pot pie

**Ingredients:**
*For the Filling:*
- 1 cup dried brown or green lentils, rinsed
- 1 tbsp olive oil
- 1 onion, diced
- 3 cloves garlic, minced
- 2 carrots, peeled and diced
- 2 celery stalks, diced
- 8 oz mushrooms, sliced
- 2 cups vegetable broth
- 1 tsp dried thyme
- 1 tsp dried rosemary
- Salt and pepper to taste

*For the Crust:*
- 1 1/2 cups all-purpose flour
- 1 tsp baking powder
- 1/2 tsp salt
- 6 tbsp cold unsalted butter, cubed
- 1/4 cup ice water

**Instructions:**

1. Preheat oven to 400°F.

2. In a large pot, cover the lentils with water and bring to a boil. Reduce heat and simmer for 15-20 minutes until tender. Drain and set aside.

3. In the same pot, heat the olive oil over medium heat. Add the onion, garlic, carrots, celery and mushrooms. Sauté for 5-7 minutes until vegetables are softened.

4. Stir in the cooked lentils, vegetable broth, thyme, rosemary, salt and pepper. Simmer for 10 minutes.

5. Transfer the lentil and vegetable filling to a 9-inch pie dish.

6. Make the crust: In a food processor, pulse the flour, baking powder and salt. Add the cold butter and pulse until mixture resembles coarse crumbs. Slowly add the ice water and pulse just until dough starts to come together.

7. Roll out the dough on a lightly floured surface to a 12-inch circle. Place the dough over the filling and crimp the edges to seal.

8. Cut a few slits in the top of the crust to allow steam to escape. Bake for 30-35 minutes, until the crust is golden brown. Let the pot pie cool for 10 minutes before serving.

This hearty lentil and vegetable filling is topped with a flaky homemade pie crust for a delicious vegetarian main dish. Enjoy!

# 90. Stuffed tomatoes with quinoa and black beans

**Ingredients:**
- 6 large tomatoes
- 1 cup cooked quinoa
- 1 (15oz) can black beans, drained and rinsed
- 1/2 cup diced onion
- 2 cloves garlic, minced
- 1 tsp ground cumin
- 1 tsp dried oregano
- Salt and pepper to taste
- Shredded cheese (optional)
- Chopped fresh basil or parsley for garnish

**Instructions**:

1. Preheat oven to 375°F.

2. Slice the tops off the tomatoes and scoop out the insides, leaving a 1/4-inch shell. Finely chop the tomato insides.

3. In a bowl, mix together the chopped tomato insides, cooked quinoa, black beans, onion, garlic, cumin, oregano, salt and pepper.

4. Stuff the quinoa and black bean mixture into the hollowed out tomato shells.

5. If desired, top the stuffed tomatoes with shredded cheese.

6. Place the stuffed tomatoes in a baking dish. Bake for 20-25 minutes, until the tomatoes are tender.

7. Remove from oven and garnish with chopped fresh basil or parsley.

8. Serve the stuffed tomatoes warm.

The combination of quinoa, black beans, and aromatic spices makes a delicious and nutritious filling for the fresh tomato shells. The cheese topping is optional but adds a nice creamy element.

***These stuffed tomatoes make a great vegetarian main dish or side. You can adjust the seasonings to your taste.***

# 91. Tofu and vegetable pad Thai

**Ingredients:**
- 8 oz rice noodles
- 2 tbsp vegetable oil
- 1 block extra-firm tofu, pressed and cubed
- 2 cloves garlic, minced
- 1 cup shredded carrots
- 1 cup bean sprouts
- 1 cup chopped broccoli florets
- 2 eggs, lightly beaten
- 3 tbsp tamarind paste
- 2 tbsp fish sauce (or soy sauce for vegan)
- 1 tbsp brown sugar
- 1 lime, cut into wedges
- Chopped peanuts, cilantro and crushed red pepper flakes for serving

**Instructions:**

1. Soak the rice noodles in hot water for 15-20 minutes until softened. Drain and set aside.

2. In a large skillet or wok, heat the vegetable oil over medium-high heat. Add the tofu cubes and cook for 2-3 minutes per side until lightly browned. Remove tofu from pan and set aside.

3. In the same pan, add the garlic, carrots, bean sprouts and broccoli. Stir-fry for 3-4 minutes until vegetables are tender-crisp.

4. Push the vegetables to the side of the pan and pour in the beaten eggs. Scramble the eggs for 1-2 minutes until cooked through.

5. Add the cooked rice noodles, tofu, tamarind paste, fish sauce and brown sugar. Toss everything together until well combined and heated through.

6. Remove from heat and squeeze fresh lime juice over the pad thai.

7. Serve the tofu and vegetable pad thai immediately, garnished with chopped peanuts, cilantro and crushed red pepper flakes.

**The combination of chewy rice noodles, crispy tofu, fresh veggies and the sweet-tangy pad thai sauce makes this a delicious and satisfying vegetarian dish. Adjust the seasonings to your taste.**

# 92. Stuffed mushrooms with quinoa and black beans

**Ingredients:**
- 12 large mushrooms, stems removed and chopped
- 1 tbsp olive oil
- 1 small onion, diced
- 2 cloves garlic, minced
- 1 cup cooked quinoa
- 1 (15oz) can black beans, drained and rinsed
- 1/4 cup grated Parmesan cheese
- 1 tsp dried oregano
- Salt and pepper to taste
- Chopped parsley for garnish

**Instructions:**

1. Preheat oven to 375°F. Arrange the mushroom caps, gill-side up, on a baking sheet.

2. In a skillet, heat the olive oil over medium heat. Add the chopped mushroom stems, onion and garlic. Sauté for 3-4 minutes until softened.

3. Stir in the cooked quinoa, black beans, Parmesan cheese, oregano, salt and pepper. Mix well.

4. Spoon the quinoa and black bean mixture evenly into the mushroom caps.

5. Bake for 15-20 minutes, until the mushrooms are tender.

6. Remove from oven and garnish the stuffed mushrooms with chopped parsley.

7. Serve the stuffed mushrooms warm.

The earthy mushrooms pair perfectly with the protein-packed quinoa and black beans. The Parmesan cheese adds a nice savory flavor to the filling.

These stuffed mushrooms make a great vegetarian appetizer or side dish. You can adjust the amount of oregano or add other herbs to suit your taste.

*Enjoy these flavorful and nutritious stuffed mushrooms!*

# 93. Tofu and vegetable sushi bowl

**Ingredients**:
- 2 cups cooked sushi rice
- 1 block extra-firm tofu, pressed and cubed
- 1 cup shredded carrots
- 1 cup shredded cucumber
- 1 cup shredded red cabbage
- 1/2 cup edamame, shelled
- 2 scallions, sliced
- 2 tbsp rice vinegar
- 1 tbsp soy sauce
- 1 tsp sesame oil
- 1 tsp sesame seeds
- Salt and pepper to taste
- Pickled ginger, for serving (optional)

**Instructions:**

1. In a large bowl, combine the cooked sushi rice, tofu cubes, shredded carrots, cucumber, red cabbage, edamame and sliced scallions.

2. In a small bowl, whisk together the rice vinegar, soy sauce, sesame oil and sesame seeds.

3. Drizzle the vinegar-soy dressing over the sushi bowl and gently toss to coat.

4. Season the sushi bowl with salt and pepper to taste.

5. Serve the tofu and vegetable sushi bowl immediately, garnished with pickled ginger if desired.

The combination of warm sushi rice, crisp veggies, protein-rich tofu, and the tangy-sweet dressing creates a delicious and satisfying sushi bowl.

You can customize the ingredients based on your preferences - try adding avocado, mushrooms, or other favorite sushi fillings.

***This makes a great vegetarian main dish or side. Enjoy this fresh and flavorful sushi bowl!***

# 94. Vegan bibimbap bowl

**Ingredients:**
- 1 cup cooked brown rice
- 1 cup shredded carrots
- 1 cup shredded spinach
- 1 cup sliced mushrooms
- 1 cup bean sprouts
- 1 avocado, sliced
- 2 tbsp gochujang (Korean chili paste)
- 2 tbsp soy sauce
- 1 tsp sesame oil
- 1 tsp sesame seeds
- Salt and pepper to taste
- Chopped scallions for garnish

**Instructions:**

1. In a large bowl, layer the cooked brown rice, shredded carrots, spinach, sliced mushrooms, and bean sprouts.

2. Top the bibimbap bowl with sliced avocado.

3. In a small bowl, whisk together the gochujang, soy sauce, sesame oil and sesame seeds to make the bibimbap sauce.

4. Drizzle the gochujang sauce over the bibimbap bowl.

5. Season the bowl with salt and pepper to taste.

6. Garnish the vegan bibimbap with chopped scallions.

7. Serve the bibimbap bowl warm, mixing everything together before eating.

This colorful and flavorful vegan bibimbap is packed with nutritious vegetables, creamy avocado, and a delicious gochujang sauce. The combination of textures and flavors makes it a satisfying meatless meal.

You can adjust the vegetables based on your preferences. The gochujang sauce provides a tasty Korean-inspired kick.

***This makes a great vegan main dish or side. Enjoy!***

# 95. Lentil and vegetable biryani

**Ingredients:**
- 1 cup dried brown or green lentils, rinsed
- 2 tbsp ghee or vegetable oil
- 1 onion, diced
- 3 cloves garlic, minced
- 1 tbsp grated fresh ginger
- 2 tsp garam masala
- 1 tsp ground cumin
- 1 tsp ground coriander
- 1/2 tsp turmeric
- 1/4 tsp cayenne pepper (optional)
- 1 cup diced tomatoes
- 1 cup vegetable broth
- 1 medium potato, peeled and cubed
- 1 cup cauliflower florets
- 1 cup frozen peas
- 1 cup basmati rice
- Chopped cilantro for garnish
- Yogurt or raita, for serving (optional)

**Instructions:**

1. In a medium saucepan, cover the lentils with water and bring to a boil. Reduce heat and simmer for 15-20 minutes until tender. Drain and set aside.

2. In a large skillet or Dutch oven, heat the ghee or oil over medium heat. Add the onion and sauté for 5 minutes until translucent.

3. Stir in the garlic, ginger, garam masala, cumin, coriander, turmeric and cayenne (if using). Cook for 1 minute until fragrant.

4. Add the diced tomatoes, vegetable broth, potato, cauliflower and peas. Bring to a simmer.

5. Stir in the cooked lentils and basmati rice. Cover and cook for 15-20 minutes, until the rice is tender.

6. Remove from heat and let stand, covered, for 5 minutes.

7. Fluff the lentil biryani with a fork. Garnish with chopped cilantro.

8. Serve the lentil and vegetable biryani warm, with yogurt or raita on the side if desired.

**The blend of aromatic spices creates a delicious Indian-inspired biryani. The lentils and vegetables make it a hearty and nutritious vegetarian main dish. Adjust the spices to your preference.**

# 96. Vegetable curry with seitan

**Ingredients:**
- 1 tbsp coconut oil
- 1 onion, diced
- 3 cloves garlic, minced
- 1 tbsp grated fresh ginger
- 2 tsp garam masala
- 1 tsp ground cumin
- 1 tsp ground coriander
- 1/2 tsp turmeric
- 1/4 tsp cayenne pepper (optional)
- 1 (14oz) can diced tomatoes
- 1 cup vegetable broth
- 1 medium potato, peeled and cubed
- 1 cup cauliflower florets
- 1 cup green beans, trimmed and cut into 1-inch pieces
- 8 oz seitan, cubed
- 1 (13.5oz) can coconut milk
- Salt and pepper to taste
- Chopped cilantro for garnish

**Instructions:**

1. In a large skillet or Dutch oven, heat the coconut oil over medium heat. Add the onion and sauté for 5 minutes until translucent.

2. Stir in the garlic, ginger, garam masala, cumin, coriander, turmeric and cayenne (if using). Cook for 1 minute until fragrant.

3. Add the diced tomatoes, vegetable broth, potato, cauliflower and green beans. Bring to a simmer.

4. Add the cubed seitan and coconut milk. Simmer for 15-20 minutes, until the vegetables are tender.

5. Season the curry with salt and pepper to taste.

6. Serve the vegetable curry with seitan warm, garnished with chopped cilantro. Can be served over rice or with naan bread.

The combination of aromatic spices, creamy coconut milk, and hearty seitan makes this a delicious and satisfying vegetarian curry. Adjust the amount of cayenne to control the heat level.

**Seitan provides a meaty texture, but you can substitute extra vegetables or chickpeas if preferred. Enjoy this flavorful curry!**

# 97. Stuffed bell peppers with lentils and bulgur

**Ingredients:**
- 6 bell peppers (any color)
- 1 cup cooked lentils
- 1 cup cooked bulgur
- 1 small onion, diced
- 2 cloves garlic, minced
- 1 cup diced tomatoes
- 1 tsp ground cumin
- 1 tsp dried oregano
- Salt and pepper to taste
- Shredded cheese (optional)

**Instructions:**
1. Preheat oven to 375°F.

2. Cut the tops off the bell peppers and remove the seeds and membranes. Place the peppers in a baking dish.

3. In a bowl, combine the cooked lentils, bulgur, onion, garlic, diced tomatoes, cumin, oregano, salt and pepper.

4. Stuff the lentil and bulgur mixture into the hollowed out bell peppers.

5. If desired, top the stuffed peppers with shredded cheese.

6. Bake for 30-35 minutes, until the peppers are tender.

7. Serve the stuffed bell peppers warm.

The lentils and bulgur provide a hearty, fiber-rich filling for the bell peppers. The tomatoes, onion and spices add great flavor. You can adjust the seasonings to your taste.

Bulgur is a quick-cooking whole grain that pairs nicely with the lentils in this recipe. The cheese topping is optional but adds a nice creamy element.

***These stuffed peppers make a delicious and nutritious vegetarian main dish. Serve them with a side salad or roasted vegetables for a complete meal.***

# 98. Tofu and vegetable stir-fry with almonds

**Ingredients:**
- 1 block (14 oz) extra-firm tofu, cubed
- 2 tbsp vegetable oil
- 1 red bell pepper, sliced
- 1 cup broccoli florets
- 1 cup sliced mushrooms
- 1 cup snow peas or snap peas
- 3 cloves garlic, minced
- 1 tbsp grated ginger
- 2 tbsp soy sauce
- 1 tbsp rice vinegar
- 1 tsp sesame oil
- 1/4 cup roasted sliced almonds

**Instructions**:

1. Press the tofu for 15-30 minutes to remove excess moisture. Cut into 1-inch cubes.

2. Heat the vegetable oil in a large skillet or wok over high heat. Add the tofu and cook for 2-3 minutes per side until lightly browned. Remove tofu from pan and set aside.

3. Add the bell pepper, broccoli, mushrooms and snow peas to the pan. Stir-fry for 3-4 minutes until vegetables are tender-crisp.

4. Add the garlic and ginger and cook for 1 minute until fragrant.

5. Return the tofu to the pan. Add the soy sauce, rice vinegar and sesame oil. Toss everything together and cook for 2-3 more minutes.

6. Remove from heat and stir in the roasted sliced almonds. Serve the tofu and vegetable stir-fry immediately over rice or noodles.

The combination of crispy tofu, fresh vegetables and crunchy almonds makes this a delicious and nutritious stir-fry. Adjust the sauce ingredients to your taste.

**The almonds add a nice nutty flavor and texture to the dish. Feel free to substitute other nuts if desired.**

# 99. Chickpea and vegetable tagine

**Ingredients:**
- 2 tbsp olive oil
- 1 onion, diced
- 3 cloves garlic, minced
- 1 tsp ground cumin
- 1 tsp ground coriander
- 1 tsp paprika
- 1/2 tsp ground cinnamon
- 1/4 tsp cayenne pepper (optional)
- 1 (15oz) can chickpeas, drained and rinsed
- 1 (14oz) can diced tomatoes
- 1 cup vegetable broth
- 1 medium sweet potato, peeled and cubed
- 1 cup cauliflower florets
- 1 cup green beans, trimmed and cut into 1-inch pieces
- Salt and pepper to taste
- Chopped cilantro for garnish

**Instructions:**
1. In a large pot or Dutch oven, heat the olive oil over medium heat. Add the onion and sauté for 5 minutes until translucent.

2. Add the garlic, cumin, coriander, paprika, cinnamon and cayenne (if using). Cook for 1 minute until fragrant.

3. Stir in the chickpeas, diced tomatoes, vegetable broth, sweet potato, cauliflower and green beans. Season with salt and pepper.

4. Bring the mixture to a simmer, then reduce heat to medium-low. Cover and cook for 20-25 minutes, until the vegetables are tender.

5. Taste and adjust seasonings as needed. Serve the chickpea and vegetable tagine warm, garnished with chopped cilantro. Can be served over couscous or rice.

The blend of spices creates a delicious Moroccan-inspired flavor in this hearty vegetable and chickpea stew. Feel free to substitute other vegetables as desired.

**The chickpeas provide protein and fiber to make this a satisfying vegetarian main dish. Adjust the amount of cayenne to control the heat level.**

# 100. Stuffed sweet potatoes with lentils and quinoa

**Ingredients:**
- 4 medium sweet potatoes
- 1 cup cooked lentils
- 1 cup cooked quinoa
- 1 cup diced tomatoes
- 1 small onion, diced
- 2 cloves garlic, minced
- 1 tsp ground cumin
- 1 tsp chili powder
- Salt and pepper to taste
- Chopped cilantro for garnish
- Shredded cheese (optional)

**Instructions:**
1. Preheat oven to 400°F. Pierce the sweet potatoes several times with a fork. Bake for 45-60 minutes, until very soft when squeezed.

2. Let the sweet potatoes cool slightly, then slice them in half lengthwise. Scoop out the flesh into a bowl, leaving a thin layer attached to the skin.

3. In the bowl with the sweet potato flesh, mix together the cooked lentils, quinoa, diced tomatoes, onion, garlic, cumin, chili powder, salt and pepper.

4. Stuff the sweet potato skins with the lentil and quinoa mixture.

5. Place the stuffed sweet potatoes on a baking sheet. Bake for 10-15 minutes, until heated through.

6. Remove from oven and top with chopped cilantro and shredded cheese, if desired. Serve warm.

The combination of sweet potatoes, lentils, quinoa and vegetables makes these stuffed sweet potatoes a nutritious and flavorful vegetarian main dish. The lentils and quinoa provide protein and fiber.

You can adjust the spices to your taste. The cheese topping is optional but adds a nice creamy element.

***These make a great meatless meal or side dish. Enjoy!***

*As you reach the end of **"100+ Vegan Recipes for Managing Diverticulitis Flare-Ups,"** we hope you feel empowered and inspired to take control of your health through delicious, plant-based meals. Throughout this journey, we've explored the intersection of vegan cuisine and digestive wellness, offering a diverse array of recipes designed to support individuals living with diverticulitis.*

*Managing diverticulitis can be a challenging endeavor, but by prioritizing wholesome, gut-friendly ingredients, we can alleviate symptoms, promote healing, and enhance overall well-being. Whether you've been following a vegan lifestyle for years or are just beginning to explore plant-based eating, we hope you've discovered new favorites and gained valuable insights into nourishing your body with compassion and intention.*

*As you continue on your journey, remember that food is not only sustenance but also a source of joy, connection, and healing. Experiment with flavors, embrace seasonal ingredients, and listen to your body's unique needs as you craft meals that nourish both body and soul.*

*We extend our heartfelt gratitude to you for choosing this cookbook as a companion on your path to wellness. May these recipes bring warmth to your kitchen, comfort to your belly, and vitality to your life. Here's to vibrant health, delicious food, and thriving with diverticulitis. Bon appétit!*